YIN & YANG

A Practical Guide to Eating A Balanced & Healthy Diet

Oliver Cowmeadow

Cornish Connection

Fifth Edition September 1992
ISBN 0 948603 00 3
© Oliver Cowmeadow 1985

Published by Cornish Connection
The Coach House, Buckyette Farm, Littlehempston,
Totnes, Devon TQ9 6ND

Typeset and printed by Gorsefield Graphics
Roche, St Austell, Cornwall PL26 8HX

Contents

Introduction

Over the last few decades many people have become aware that the way we eat has a big effect on our physical health, and on our emotions and behaviour. This has led to a wide-spread reassessment of what constitutes a healthy diet, and the publishing of hundreds of books proposing the benefits of a wide range of diets. Some of these diets are based on a single idea, such as eating raw foods, or eating more fibre, and lack a comprehensive understanding of what constitutes a healthy diet. Others take an analytical approach, involving the counting of calories and other food components, which can be difficult to apply to daily eating. Few consider how our diet should be changed to suit different environments and varying individual needs.

The beauty of applying yin and yang to diet is that the principles are easy to understand and apply, and also to relate to other aspects of our lives. They make it simple to understand the connection between our diet, various physical ailments, and our emotions and attitudes, and also how to adapt our diet to differences in climate, season and personal needs.

Through eating a diet in which yin and yang are balanced, we produce harmony and equilibrium within us, and between ourselves and our environment. Physiologically this is experienced as health, and physiologically it is experienced as happiness. Every individual's experience of restoring balance will be different according to their state of health and personal character, but for everyone it is the path to a more peaceful, happy and enjoyable life.

Yin and Yang

The words yin and yang come from Japan, but the universal occurrence of these two tendencies was once recognised by people worldwide, including the Celts, early Greek philosophers and Christians, ancient Egyptians, Incas and North American Indians. Yin and yang are the two tendencies or forces that produce all the pairs of opposites that are found everywhere in our relative world. This includes hot and cold, summer and winter, acid and alkaline, positive and negative electric and magnetic poles, male and female, the sodium/potassium balance within our bodies, and opposite emotions, attitudes and psychological states.

Everything is formed by both the yin and yang tendencies, nothing is solely yin or yang. They combine in varying proportions to create all forms and phenomena.

The yang tendency is of compaction, and can be represented by a centripetal spiral -

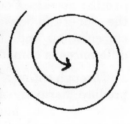

This compaction produces greater activity, and also heat as when air is compressed pumping up a tyre, and the warm colours red, orange and yellow. When the yang force predominates it forms smaller and harder objects with a greater density and weight.

The yin tendency is of expansion, and can be represented by a centrifugal spiral -

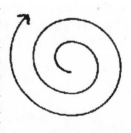

Expansion produces more inactivity, and coolness as can be felt when expanding gas is released from an aerosol can, and the cooler colours green, blue and violet. When the yin tendency predominates larger and softer objects are formed with less density and weight.

On Earth the yang force comes from the sun, moon, planets, stars and outer space in the form of light, other electromagnetic radiations, and cosmic rays, moving to the Earth's centre. The yin force is produced by the rotation of the Earth, and expands from its centre outwards. Therefore at the surface of the Earth where we live, the yang force moves downwards, and the yin force moves upwards. Here the intense interaction of the two forces produces and sustains life.

In the northern hemisphere the yang tendency, which may be called heaven's force, moves in an anticlockwise spiral. These directions are reversed in the southern hemisphere.

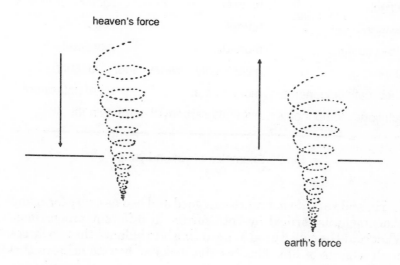

Fig. 1. The direction of yin and yang at the earth's surface.

These examples of yin and yang are summarised in the table below, together with some further indications of the yin and yang nature of foods.

Quality	Yang	Yin
Movement	centripetal	centrifugal
Direction	downwards	upwards
Temperature	warmer	colder
Colour	red - orange - yellow - green - blue - violet	
Size	small	large
Density	more dense	less dense
Weight	heavier	lighter
Texture	harder	softer
Water content	more dry	more wet
Taste	bitter - salty - sweet - sour - pungent	
Chemical components	more sodium	more potassium
Nutritional components	minerals-carbohydrate-protein-fat-oil	

Fig.2. Examples of yin and yang.

Yin and yang do not represent good and bad as every form and phenomena is formed by both forces, in different proportions. What could be called good or desirable is to balance the two forces in all aspects of life. This booklet looks at how to achieve this balance in our diet, which will produce physical health and emotional and mental balance, helping to create a peaceful, creative and fulfilling life.

Yin and Yang in the Plant World

The structure of plants clearly shows how yin and yang create different forms. A sprouting seed on the surface of the ground sends a root downwards and a leafy shoot upwards. The root is formed more by the descending and contracting yang force, and so becomes compact and hard, often with a red or orange colour. The shoot is formed more by the ascending and expanding yin force, producing the green expanded leaves. In this way all the vegetables that we eat can be classified on a scale from yang to yin.

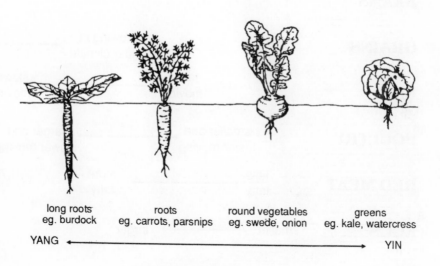

| long roots | roots | round vegetables | greens |
| eg. burdock | eg. carrots, parsnips | eg. swede, onion | eg. kale, watercress |

YANG ⟵――――――――――――――――――――⟶ YIN

Fig. 3. Vegetables arranged from yang to yin.

The Yin and Yang of Food

Using the criteria given above, all of our foods can be classified on a scale from yang to yin, as in the table on the next two pages.

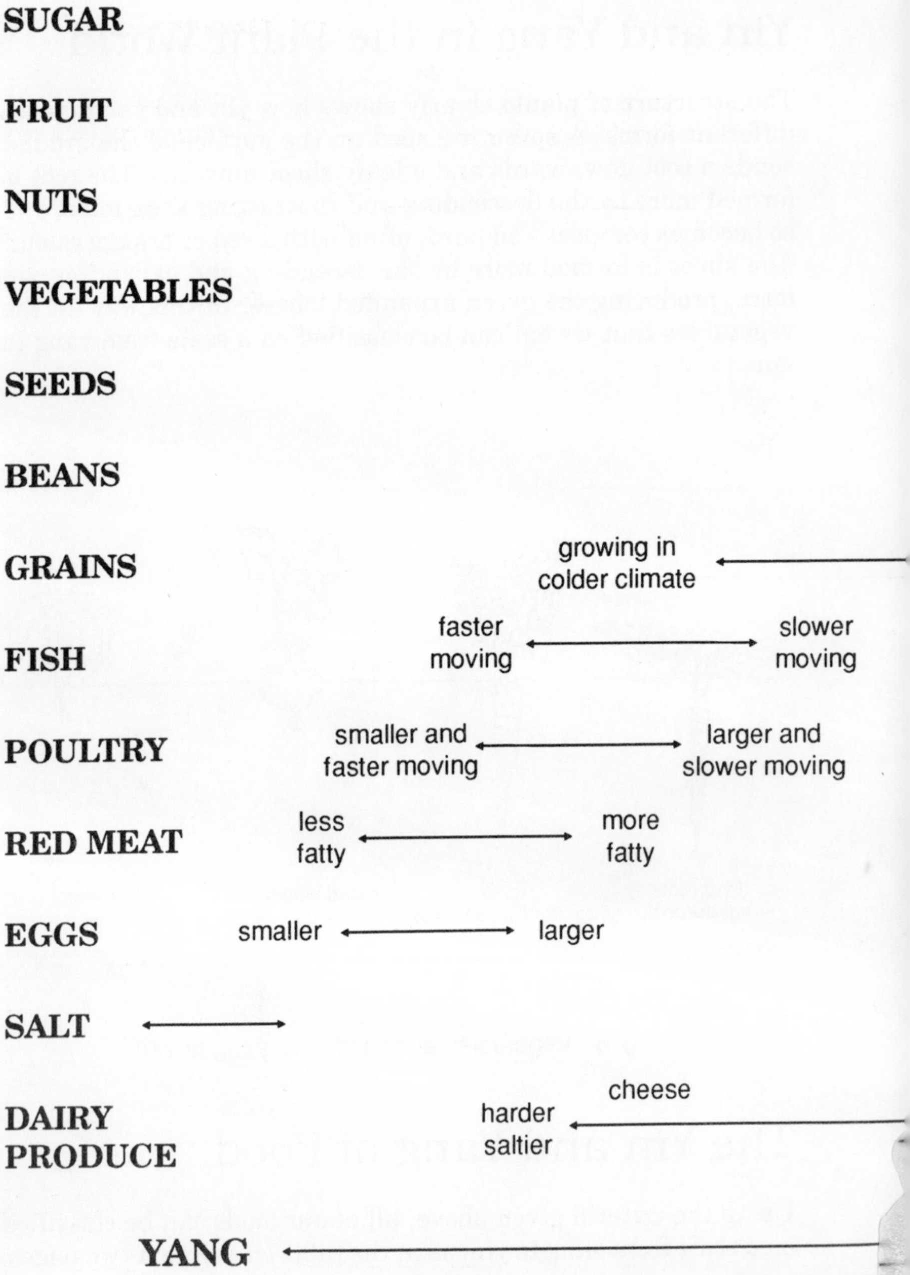

SUGAR

FRUIT

NUTS

VEGETABLES

SEEDS

BEANS

GRAINS
growing in
colder climate ←

faster   slower
FISH   moving ←————————→ moving

smaller and ←————————→ larger and
POULTRY   faster moving   slower moving

less ←————————→ more
RED MEAT   fatty   fatty

EGGS   smaller ←————————→ larger

SALT ←————————→

cheese
harder ←—————
DAIRY   saltier
PRODUCE

YANG ←————————————————————

Fig 4. A classification

8

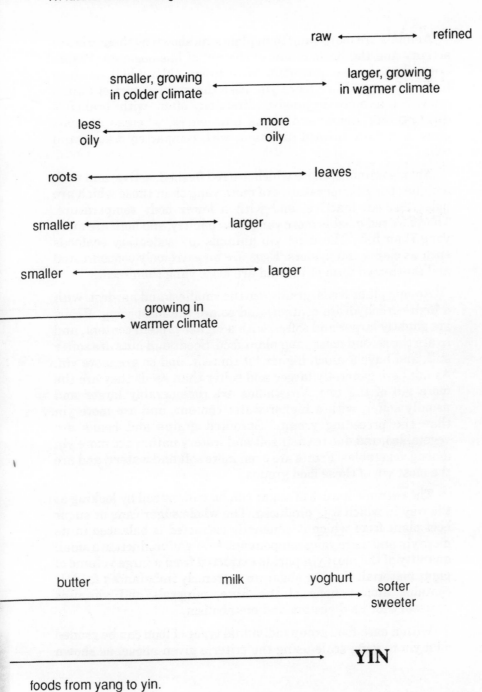

raw ←————————→ refined

smaller, growing
in colder climate ←————————→ larger, growing
in warmer climate

less
oily ←————————→ more
oily

roots ←————————————→ leaves

smaller ←————————→ larger

smaller ←————————————→ larger

————————→ growing in
warmer climate

butter   milk   yoghurt
                                                    softer
sweeter

————————————————————————→ **YIN**

foods from yang to yin.

Animals are more yang than plants, as shown by their greater activity and the basic colour of the red of haemoglobin. Plants are sedentary and immobile, with green chlorophyll as their basic colour, and are more yin. Also the greater part of plants grows in a more expansive direction, often with branches dividing into stems, and stems into leaves, whereas animals grow in a more inward direction, with compacted organs and cells.

Among animals, those which are red fleshed, active, and with a higher body temperature are more yang than those which are paler fleshed, inactive, and with a lower body temperature. Therefore red meat is more yang than poultry, and both are more yang than fish. The most yin animals are sedentary seafoods such as clams and oysters. Eggs are an extremely concentrated and contracted form of life and are more yang than meats.

Among plant foods, grains are the smallest and hardest, with a high carbohydrate content, and so are the most yang. Beans are slightly larger and softer, with a higher protein content, and so are the second most yang plant food. Seeds and nuts are softer still, and have a much higher fat content, and so are more yin. As nuts are generally larger and softer than seeds they are the more yin of the two. Vegetables are considerably larger and usually softer, with a higher water content, and are more yin than the preceding groups. Sprouted grains and beans are vegetables, and due to their soft and watery nature are more yin among vegetables. Fruits are even more soft and watery, and are the most yin of these food groups.

The extreme nature of sugar can be understood by looking at the way in which it is produced. The whole sugar cane or sugar beet plant from which it is usually extracted is balanced in its more yin and more yang components. In sugar production a small quantity of the most yin part is extracted from a large volume of plant material, making sugar an extremely imbalanced food. It contains almost none of the fibre, minerals and vitamins necessary for its digestion and metabolism.

Within each food group individual types of food can be graded on a yin to yang scale using the criteria given above, as shown within the vegetables in the previous section. Within the cereal grains, yang varieties are smaller, more rounded and harder, while yin varieties are larger, more elongated and softer. Arranged from yang to yin they are buckwheat, millet, short grain brown rice, wheat, barley, oats, and corn. There are different varieties of some grains which can also be arranged from yang to yin, for example rice, in which the order is short grain, medium grain, and long grain. Among the beans the smaller varieties containing less oil, for example aduki beans, are more yang than larger beans that contain more oil, such as butter beans. The same is true for nuts, with smaller and less oily varieties being more yang, and larger and more oily types being more yin. You can work out how to arrange the foods within the other groups using the general characteristics of yin and yang foods. You can also use the season and climate in which a plant grows after reading further sections of this book.

In recent years man's activities and methods of agriculture and food production have made the average diet of a more extreme nature. Artificial chemicals such as food additives, drugs and medications, as well as various forms of radiation, are far more yin than sugar and have a very extreme effect on our body and mental state. The refining of a food generally makes it more yin by removing fibre and minerals, and often producing a more soft and watery texture. The use of nitrates and other fertilisers creates larger plants, which are more yin, often containing less minerals and more water. You may well have noticed that smaller vegetables often have much more flavour than larger ones.

A Balanced Diet

When we eat, the energy of the food and our energy merge together - after eating we have become a new person. Most of the atoms and cells of our body have come from the food that we have eaten. There is much truth in the old saying, "we are what we eat". Before reading on, think of the different qualities of the foods that you eat, and decide which you would like to become and those that you would not like to become.

We can get a clearer understanding of the effects of different foods on us by using yin and yang. If we eat predominantly yang foods we become more yang, and if we eat more of the yin foods we become more yin. In either case the imbalance in our condition will produce problems. To achieve a balance at every level of our being it is necessary to eat a diet with yin and yang foods in balance with each other.

The yin and yang forces naturally move to create balance in the universe and in ourselves, so we intuitively make a crude balance in our choice of foods. For example, spicy sauces are favourites on eggs and sausages; salad and pickles are usually eaten with cheese; we feel attracted to fruit, sugar or alcohol after eating meat; bread, a dry and hard preparation of grains, is eaten with oily and sugary spreads. However the combination of these extreme yang and extreme yin foods cannot create balance, as their individual effects are too strong, with some organs and systems in the body becoming over-expanded and others becoming over contracted.

To achieve balance in our condition we need to make up our diet from the foods centrally placed on the yin - yang scale. Within this narrower range a balance can be maintained between the more yin and more yang foods. In general whole cereal grains can provide us with the more yang qualities that we need, and should form about half of our diet, as they have in most advanced cultures and civilisations over past millennia. These can be balanced by making up the other half of the diet with the more yin food groups of vegetables, beans, seeds, nuts and fruit, in the proportions shown in figure 5 below.

This diagram represents the proportions to be eaten over one day. An individual meal could contain only one or two of the food groups, as long as the other groups are included at other meals the same day to make up the correct proportions. Due to the balanced nature of the cereal grains, they should generally be included in every meal.

This diet plan is generally suitable for all people living in a temperate climate with four distinct seasons, such as in Great Britain and other northern European countries, and North

America. It needs to be modified for people living in polar or tropical climates, over the changing seasons, and to suit differing personal needs, as will be described later.

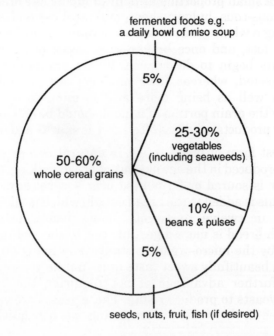

Fig. 5. A diet balanced in its yin and yang foods.

In planning a balanced diet, as well as considering the qualities of different foods, it is important to consider the quantities in which they are eaten. No food can be said to be good for the health in any quantity, as this ignores the idea of balance. For example, if too large a proportion of grains are eaten, one becomes too yang, with too much carbohydrate and minerals in the body and not enough protein and oil. Excessive quantities of beans will make one too yin, with an excess of protein. If large amounts of fruit are eaten one will also become imbalanced with a yin condition, and an excess of fluid. Scientific analysis has shown that when the foods are eaten in the proportions shown in figure 5 the diet contains plentiful amounts of all essential nutrients, including protein, essential oils, and the different

13

minerals and vitamins.

The cereal grains should be eaten mainly in their whole form, with only a small proportion as flour products like bread, pastry, noodles, cous-cous, bulgar wheat, and steel cut and rolled oats. In splitting a whole grain into many fragments much of its vital charge is lost, and once broken open some of its nutritional components begin to decompose. Whole grains are also very easily digested, whereas flour products are more difficult to digest, as well as being more acid forming in the stomach. Generally the grain portion of a meal should be of whole grains, with flour products used less often and as snacks and in desserts.

The best form of bread to eat is natural rise or sourdough, which is produced in the age old way of bread making. Some flour and water is soured or fermented over several days to form a starter. This is added to the bread dough, which is allowed to rise naturally in twelve to twenty hours before being baked. Sourdough bread is more digestible due to the 'pre-digestion' of the flour by the micro-organisms naturally living on grains. It also has a beautifully sweet taste quite unlike yeasted bread. It has the further advantage of not requiring the addition of artificial yeasts to produce rising. These yeasts are very yin, as can be seen in their effect of producing the very quick rising of breads.

The vegetable portion of the diet should contain root, round and leafy varieties so that a balance is achieved between yin and yang within the vegetables. This can include a small amount of seaweeds, such as kombu (kelp), wakame, dulse, arame, hiziki, Irish moss, nori and agar agar, to make up about 3% of the whole diet. They provide a very rich source of minerals such as calcium and iron, and also vitamin A. Some types can be used in soups, such as dulse and wakame, others can be prepared as separate dishes, for example arame and hiziki. Kombu can be cooked in stews and with beans, and the flat sheets of nori can be used to wrap around balls of rice or cut into thin strips as a garnish for soups. Agar-agar is a setting agent used in making jellies and moulds.

Seaweeds growing in a water environment have a

fundamentally different quality compared with land vegetables growing in an air environment. This can be understood by realising that water is more yang than air, and that the plants produced in a certain environment have an opposite and complimentary nature to their surroundings. Therefore plants growing in the more yang water are more yin in form, and those growing in the more yin air are more yang. Thus seaweeds are generally more expanded and flexible, whereas land plants are more compacted with a more rigid structure. Therefore the seaweeds form a more yin part of the vegetable portion of the diet.

Beans and pulses provide a rich source of vegetable protein that is easily digested and assimilated by the body, as well as high levels of some minerals and vitamins such as calcium, iron and vitamin B. Due to their high protein content, and in some types also high oil content, they are ideally cooked with a small amount of mineral rich seaweed like wakame or kelp. This creates a more balanced food that is easier to digest and utilise in the body.

Traditionally made fermented foods are a useful part of the diet as a source of vitamin B_{12} (otherwise only obtainable from animal foods), and enzymes beneficial to digestion. This includes vegetables pickled with salt, for example sauerkraut, umeboshi (green plums pickled in sea salt), traditionally brewed beers and other beverages, shoyu (a good quality soy sauce), and miso. Shoyu and miso are traditionally produced by the slow fermentation of soya beans and different cereal grains such as barley, wheat or rice, together with sea salt, over a period longer than one and a half years. Miso is in the form of a paste, and is primarily used to give a rich flavour to soups, stews, sauces and other dishes. Shoyu is in a liquid form, and can be used instead of salt to flavour a wide variety of dishes, including vegetables, beans, and soups. Fermented foods should form about 5% of the diet, which could be made up of a daily bowl of soup seasoned with miso or shoyu, the regular use of pickled vegetables, and the occasional brewed beverage if desired.

Seeds, nuts and fruit form 3-5% of the diet. Seeds and nuts are preferably roasted in the oven or in a dry skillet, and can be lightly seasoned with sea salt or shoyu to make the large amount of oil which they contain more balanced and digestible. They can be used as snacks or in combination with vegetables and in desserts. Fruits are the most yin of the food groups regularly consumed as part of this diet, and should therefore be eaten only two to four times a week. To make them slightly more yang they can be cooked with a small amount of salt (this also makes them sweeter).

Fish and seafood can form a small additional part of the diet, but for many people are not essential. As these are the most yang of the foods included in this diet, it is preferable to choose the more yin varieties. Among fish these are the white fleshed types, for example plaice, flounder, cod, haddock, and trout. Within seafoods the sedentary species that are more yin, for example oysters, mussels and cockles, can be eaten more often. The more yang active species such as prawns, shrimps, crab and lobster can also be eaten occasionally. To create more balanced meals a fish or seafood dish can be prepared with a small amount of a more yin flavouring such as rice vinegar, grated root ginger juice, horseradish or mustard, and should be accompanied by a large portion of greens or salad.

Various seasonings and condiments of a balanced nature can be used to add flavour and variety to meals. In cooking, shoyu and miso can be used in the place of salt to give a richer flavour. A sharp, sour taste can be obtained from brown rice vinegar, which is less acidic and yin than commercially produced vinegars. A hot or pungent taste can be added with a small amount of horseradish, mustard or grated root ginger.

Condiments for adding to your meals on the table include sesame salt (gomasio), made from a small quantity of roasted seasalt mixed with twelve to twenty times as much roasted and ground sesame seeds. Seaweeds such as wakame and kombu can be baked in an oven until crisp and then ground to a powder. Seaweed powders can also be mixed with roasted and ground sesame seeds for a less salty condiment. A small amount, say a teaspoon a day, of a condiment greatly helps the digestion of foods, however beware of over using them as you will then be consuming too much salt.

In this diet sugar can be replaced with grain sweeteners such as barley malt (malt extract) and rice syrup, which contain the more yang sugar maltose. Dried fruits and apple juice can also be used occasionally. Brown sugar, molasses and honey all contain high levels of very yin sugars, and are better avoided.

In the past few years there has been a lot of controversy over the use of salt. With yin and yang we have an accurate way of understanding its effects and deciding how much we should use. It is the most yang of all our foods, having the most powerful contractive effect. Its over use causes many problems, including the hardening of arteries and high blood pressure. The use of a small amount in cooking, but not at the table, is generally desirable to strengthen the blood and body and to aid digestion. Only enough to bring out the natural sweetness and flavour of the food should be used, meals should not taste salty. If a person has eaten a large quantity of salt in the past, they could benefit from not using any for a period.

Of all our foods salt is probably the most difficult to learn to take at the correct level. If too much salt is used you will tend to become unduly thirsty, and may retain liquid in the body, and also be attracted to over eating, especially of yin foods like fruits and sweets. Emotionally you will tend to become 'tight', that is more tense, impatient and irritable. Too little salt can produce a lack of muscle tone, with physical weakness and poor circulation. Mentally it can produce 'spaciness' and a lack of concentration and alertness. You may notice other signs of too much or too little salt, so experiment and find the level that you actually need.

Of the various kinds of salt available, seasalt is the most balanced and suitable for our consumption. Refined salt is composed almost entirely of sodium chloride, whereas seasalt also contains approximately 12% of a wide variety of additional elements, including potassium, magnesium, and iodine. We began our evolution in the ocean, and the mineral composition of our blood and body fluids still reflects the proportions of minerals in the sea. Seasalt will therefore most closely provide a natural balance of the various elements that our bodies require. As sodium is a very yang element, refined salt is also very yang. In seasalt the sodium is accompanied by more yin elements, making it a more balanced food.

Due to the yin nature of fats and oils the use of these should be small. A small amount of essential oils in the diet is necessary for health. These are primarily obtained in a balanced proportion from grains, beans, and especially from seeds and nuts. In addition a small quantity of good quality vegetable oil can be used in cooking, such as cold-pressed sesame or corn oil. One should be careful not to consume too many oily foods like margarine, and seed and nut butters like tahini and peanut butter. An excess of oils will not be burnt up, and its accumulation in the body will cause problems.

Cheese, butter, milk, yoghurt and other dairy foods should be avoided for the same reason, despite their being in the more balanced region of the yang to yin classification of foods. Common sense tells us milk is the food of babies and other newborn mammals. It provides a very rich source of nutrients necessary for rapid growth at this stage of life. The practice of consuming milk and its products is confined to only about 10% of the world's adult population of one organism, the human species. This breaking of natural law produces many problems, including the accumulation in the body of the fat from milk, which is in excess of an adult's needs. The argument that milk is necessary as a source of calcium is incorrect, as many plant foods contain more by weight, including greens like parsley, kale, and watercress, beans like chickpeas and soya beans, and especially certain seeds and seaweeds.

Beverages like coffee, commercial teas, and aromatic herb teas have a very yin nature, (as you can tell from the distance their aroma travels) and are better replaced with grain or dandelion coffee, three year twig tea (also called Bancha or Kukicha), Mu tea, or mild herb teas like chamomile. Extracting the juices of various plants involves taking the yin elements in the liquid, and leaving the more yang elements behind in the solid matter remaining. Vegetable and fruit juices are therefore more yin than the whole plant that they have been taken from. For this reason the consumption of juices should be small. In selecting juices, those from vegetables will be more yang than those from fruits, and among fruit juices those extracted from apples will be most yang.

Alcohol is more yin than water, as you can tell from its quick evaporation, and from the effects it has on you! The fermentation of different foods to produce alcoholic beverages makes those foods more yin. Beverages made from more yin foods will be more yin than those made from more yang foods. To avoid consuming excessive yin it is therefore preferable to choose types made from the most yang plants, the cereal grains, rather than those made from fruits and flowers. Small quantities of traditionally made beers, saki (rice wine), and whiskey can be drunk occasionally in reasonable quantities by those in good health, but wines and other spirits are better avoided.

Changing your eating to this balanced diet can be done progressively over a period of time. A great value of understanding the yin and yang nature of foods is that you can see which foods are the most harmful, and which are less harmful. You can begin by cutting out the most imbalanced foods, and at the same time increase your use of the more balanced foods. Red meat, eggs and sugar can be the first to reduce while increasing the use of cereal grains, beans and fresh vegetables. Later poultry, dairy foods and spices can be dropped, as you learn new ways of preparing the more balanced foods. This process can be continued at your own pace until the balanced diet is being accurately followed.

With each stage in this progression you will become more balanced, and your sensitivity to extreme foods will increase. After cutting out the more extreme foods for some time, you will probably sometimes wonder why you ever ate so much of them. This will show you that your intuitive perception of what your body actually needs is developing.

As you develop greater sensitivity to the qualities of every food you eat, you will begin to intuitively select those foods that create a healthy balance. As this sensitivity grows you can spend less time conceptually considering how to balance yin and yang in your food, and more freely eat what you feel attracted to under the guidance of your intuition.

Adapting Diet to Changing Needs

Many dietary regimes have set guidelines, irrespective of where a person lives, the prevailing climate and weather, and individual differences in constitution, present state of health, and activity. This shows a lack of understanding of the natural laws which we and all of the universe follow. To get the benefits of eating a balanced diet it is necessary to make changes in daily eating according to changing needs. What is a healthy diet for one person living in one country may be a most unhealthy diet for another individual living in a different climate with a different lifestyle. Even two people living next door to each other may need a slightly different diet according to their age, type of work, constitution and present condition. Yin and yang can guide us on how to adapt diet to these variations in the environment and between individuals. How we can do this is considered in the following sections.

Food for Different Climates

The diet of people living in different climates varies enormously, from the largely fish and meat diet of the Eskimos, to the starchy cassava and green bananas that are a staple in some regions of central Africa. How is this to be understood, will some of them become ill from consuming too much animal fat, and others from excess starch? Again this question can be understood by using the natural law of yin and yang.

In the colder, more yin polar climate the few plants that grow are much smaller and hardier, that is more yang. They contain greater amounts of minerals and fibre, more yang components of plants. In the hotter, more yang tropics plant life reaches much greater sizes, and contain more starch, oil and water, that is they are more yin. Thus plant life stays in balance with the climate they live in by evolving an opposite and complementary structure, thereby continuing in their existence from year to year.

We must also adapt to different climates to stay alive and in good health. In a polar climate a more yang diet of mostly animal foods is necessary to counter the yin cold, burning to give the body a lot of heat and energy. In the temperate climate, such as in Northern Europe or North America, little animal food is needed, and the principle foods should be the grains and vegetables growing in that climate. When living in the hot, more yang, tropical climes no animal foods are needed, and the more yin local plants with their greater cooling effect are more suitable.

Choosing a diet for living in a certain region of the world is most easily achieved by eating the foods that are traditionally grown in that locality. These plants are well adapted to that climate, so by eating them we will also become adapted to the local environment. If imported foods are eaten, these should be from a country with a similar climate. In a temperate climate such as Great Britain the grain portion of the diet can primarily be made up by short and medium grain rice, millet, wheat, barley, oats, rye, sweet brown rice, corn and buckwheat. The bean portion should can be made up of aduki beans, chickpeas and green or brown lentils, kidney, pinto, haricot, and black eye beans and split peas, including products made from soya beans like tofu, tempeh and nato.

For the vegetable part of the diet any varieties growing locally are generally suitable, but it should be noted that tomatoes, potatoes and aubergines are all tropical plants, unsuitable for us if we want to stay in balance with this climate. Although they may now be grown in temperate regions, they still retain their yin nature, as is shown by their high potassium and low sodium content.

Seeds and nuts suitable for this climate include sesame, pumpkin and sunflower seeds, and chestnuts, almonds, walnuts, hazelnuts and peanuts (which are actually a tropical bean, but are exceptionally yang due to their growth underground). Fruits can be chosen from those growing in this country, including apples, pears, apricots, cherries, peaches, strawberries, raspberries and grapes, either fresh or dried.

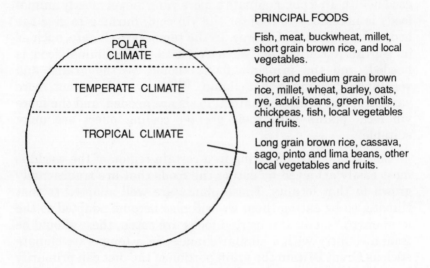

PRINCIPAL FOODS

Fish, meat, buckwheat, millet, short grain brown rice, and local vegetables.

Short and medium grain brown rice, millet, wheat, barley, oats, rye, aduki beans, green lentils, chickpeas, fish, local vegetables and fruits.

Long grain brown rice, cassava, sago, pinto and lima beans, other local vegetables and fruits.

Fig 6. Adapting diet to different climates.

With this simple and common sense understanding it can be seen that oranges are fine if you live in Morocco, but apples or strawberries are much better if you live in Britain. Brazil nuts can be enjoyed in South America, but almonds or walnuts are more suitable in Northern Europe.A lot of fish or meat is necessary if you live in the Arctic, but in a warmer temperate climate the body does not burn up all the animal fat, and so it accumulates in and around the organs causing numerous problems. However if we travel to other parts of the world, to maintain our health we must adapt our eating so that we stay in balance with the local environment. This is most easily achieved by changing to the diet traditionally eaten in the country travelled to, while keeping to the proportions given in figure 5. So a little wine can be enjoyed in Greece, a mild curry in India, and dates in Egypt!

Food for Different Seasons

We naturally feel more attracted to salads, fruits and cold drinks in the summer, and to more salty and long cooked dishes in the winter. The reason for this seems obvious, it is hotter in the summer so we are attracted to more cooling foods, and colder in the winter producing an attraction for more warming foods. To achieve a balanced condition it is necessary to have a deeper understanding of how diet should be changed over the seasons.

In the spring and summer the yang heat of the sun draws up the sap of plants, causing them to produce the yin structures of leaves and flowers. As the heat diminishes in the colder or more yin autumn and winter, the sap descends, and plants store their energy in the more yang roots and seeds. Thus as with climate, the plant world lives in harmony with the changing seasons by becoming opposite and complimentary in form.

We also need to adjust our eating through the changing seasons to stay in good health. As with plants this can be done by becoming opposite in quality to the prevailing weather. In the more yang summer months the sun tends to heat up and dehydrate us, so we need more yin cooling and watery types of food. In the more yin winter when the cold makes us shiver we require more warming or yang foods.

The easiest way to make these adjustments in diet is to follow the example of nature, and eat the seasonally available foods as they come and go over the year. Among the cereal grains, the most balanced types can be eaten all year round. The more yin and more yang grains can be eaten in larger quantities during their main season of growth and harvest, and in smaller quantities in the other seasons. Therefore short grain brown rice and wheat can form the staple grains, with buckwheat, millet, barley, oats and corn used more in the appropriate season.

The use of vegetables and fruits can follow a similar pattern. In the spring the greens that abound are ideal, and in summer lettuces, radishes, peas, green beans and the abundant summer fruits are suitable. Come the autumn we can turn to cabbages,

23

cauliflowers, pumpkins and turnips, and in winter to brussel sprouts, kale, swedes and turnips, with easily stored fruits like apples and dried fruit. Some vegetables like onions and carrots grow and can be eaten over several seasons.

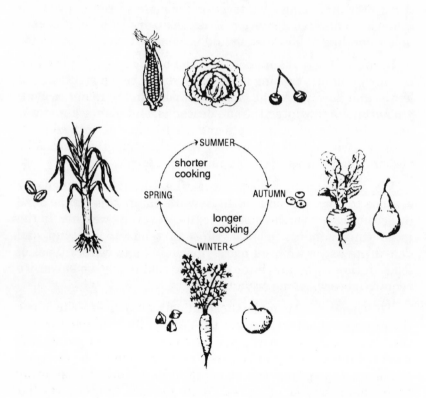

Fig. 7. Adapting diet to the seasons.

In adapting to the changing seasons, we can also use longer cooking methods with a little more salt in the autumn and winter to supply the extra heat that we need to counter the cold, and shorter cooking styles with a little less salt in the spring and summer to retain the more cooling qualities that we need in the heat.

Food for Different Individuals

Every individual differs in their age, their constitution from birth including their sex, in their present physical and psychological condition, and in their activities. Smaller personal adjustments should be made in diet to suit these differences, according to the laws of yin and yang.

As we pass through life our dietary needs change a great deal. Babies are small, compact, and very active, that is more yang. They therefore need a more yin diet for normal upward growth and development; too yang a diet will prevent this, causing stunted growth. In their first months mother's milk is obviously ideal, its liquid form reflecting its more yin nature. At weaning a diet of softened grains and other foods can be introduced, with very little salt. Harder foods can be begun when the first molars appear, with the level of salt slowly increased to the adult level by the age of seven or eight. Infants and children need a proportionately larger volume of food and drink, a larger volume or size being yin. Further information on feeding babies and children can be found in "Macrobiotic Child Care and Family Health" and other books listed in Further Reading.

On reaching adulthood a proportionately smaller volume of food is needed, with less fruit and grain sweeteners. In old age people become slightly more contracted or yang. They therefore need a slightly more yin diet, with less salt and animal food, and more lightly cooked dishes.

The biggest constitutional difference between people is their sex. The two sexes are energetically opposite and complementary to each other, with females receiving a greater proportion of the yin rising and expanding earth's force, and males receiving a greater proportion of the yang descending and contracting heaven's force. This manifests in women as a more expanded body with larger breasts, upwardly indented sexual organs, and a mental tendency to be outwardly more gentle, sensitive and receptive. In men it manifests as a taller narrower body with smaller breasts, downwardly extended sexual organs, and a mental tendency to be outwardly more active and progressive. Inwardly each sex is of the opposite tendency, so creating a harmonious balance with the outside. Women are inwardly more yang, and men are inwardly more yin.

As the constitution of the two sexes is opposite, they will need an opposite quality in their diet for each to stay in balance. Women, who are inwardly more yang, can make balance by eating a rather more yin diet. Animal foods, including fish, are less necessary for them than for men. They should generally use less salt and eat more lightly cooked dishes. Men, who are inwardly more yin, need a more yang diet. Fish can be eaten regularly if desired, and they can use some longer and stronger cooking styles, with the use of a little more salt.

When cooking for both sexes it is not necessary to cook two completely different meals! They can achieve an individual balance by choosing different proportions of the yin and yang dishes in a meal, women eating more of the yin dishes and men eating more of the yang dishes. In addition, several times a week a special dish can be prepared for only one of the sexes.

Further minor changes in diet can be made according to other differences in people's original constitution. A basic knowledge of oriental diagnosis is needed to understand these differences, which can be found in "Your Face Never Lies" and other books listed in Further Reading.

Everyone's present physical and psychological condition is different, due to the wide variety of influences that affect and form it. These include the diet eaten over one's life time up to the present moment, the amount and types of activity one does, and the particular abilities that an individual may feel they want to develop in themselves. Adjustments in diet can also be made according to these differences between individuals.

An individual's past diet will have created various physical, emotional and mental imbalances. When a person eats extreme yang foods, they will inevitably be attracted to eating some extreme yin foods to make a crude balance, and vice versa. Some people may eat roughly equal proportions of yin and yang foods, but many consume a larger proportion of either yang foods or yin foods. A person's condition may therefore fall into one of three categories, excessively yang, excessively yin, or a combination of excessively yang and yin. These conditions can be returned to a healthy balance by eating a balanced diet. This change can be accelerated by making individual dietary adjustments according to one's particular type of imbalance. If one's condition is too yang, one can eat a slightly more yin diet, if it is too yin one can eat a slightly more yang diet, and if it is a combination of the two one can eat a well balanced diet avoiding both extremes. To decide which way you have become imbalanced, read the next section on Imbalance Equals Disease, which includes dietary modifications for each direction of imbalance.

Common sense tells us that people engaged in different activities have quite different dietary requirements. More physical and social activities such as farming, labouring, public speaking, sports and business management are more yang, and require a slightly more yang diet to sustain this activity. This can be achieved with more strongly cooked and seasoned food, and more richness from vegetable sources of oil and protein, and possibly more fish. More mental, emotional, intellectual and philosophical work such as art, writing, administration, religious and spiritual activities, and social work are more yin and require a slightly more yin diet to promote these abilities. This could be achieved by using lighter cooking styles, with little or no animal foods, and a higher proportion of more yin varieties of grains and vegetables, for example barley and leafy greens. In this way you can change your eating to suit changes in your activity on a daily basis. Over a longer period of time this knowledge gives the freedom to chose those qualities and abilities that you want to develop through the selection of foods and cooking methods that promote those qualities.

Pregnancy is a time when special care is needed to ensure that the additional nutritional demands of the foetus are satisfactorily obtained in the mother's diet. Larger quantities of food rich in protein, iron, calcium and other nutrients are needed for the proper development of the child and the mother's health. At this time more beans and bean products, green leafy vegetables, seaweeds and seeds can be included in the diet. Further information on how to eat during pregnancy can be found in " Macrobiotics for Pregnancy and Care of the Newborn".

It is important to recognise how our dietary needs change on a day to day and yearly basis, and rather than stick to the same eating patterns day in, day out, to adapt the types and volume of food we take with these changing circumstances. Health is not a static state which once attained will continue indefinitely, but a continual act of maintaining an internal balance by adapting one's way of eating to changes in personal activity and environment. When beginning to eat the balanced diet, following the proportions shown in figure 5 will be enough to bring you back into balance. As your sensitivity to the effects of foods develops, you can refine your balance by adapting your eating according to changes in season, weather, your individual condition and activity on a daily basis.

The Yin and Yang of Cooking

Should we cook our food, and if so, how much? The main elements used in cooking to change the nature of the food are heat, salt, and sometimes pressure, as with pressure cooking and the pressing of pickles and salads. These influences all make for more yang, so this question is really, do we want to make our food more yang, and if so, how much?

When living in a cold climate or season, cooking is necessary to create food with a greater warming quality that generates more heat within us, making balance with the cold. In hotter climates and seasons less cooking is needed, so that some of the cooling qualities of the food are retained. In temperate climates some salads and raw foods are fine to eat in summer, but only a small quantity should be eaten in winter.Eating primarily uncooked foods during the winter will result in difficulties getting warm, chills, colds, and other more serious illnesses caused by excessive cooling of the body. There are also other good reasons for cooking certain types of food, for example to make them more digestible, as with grains, beans, and fish.

Diets with a large proportion of raw foods, some including much fruits, have recently become popular. The reason for this is easily understood using yin and yang. An attraction for uncooked foods, which are more yin, is due to the consumption of yang foods, such as meat, eggs, cheese and excessive amounts of salt, which have been consumed in increasingly large quantities in the past few decades. Wanting more yin foods is an intuitive act to restore balance. However these more extreme yang and yin foods will not create a healthy balanced state in the body.

It is often said that cooking destroys the vitamins and minerals in foods. However minerals cannot be destroyed at the temperatures used in cooking, and the only vitamin that can be broken down by normal cooking is vitamin C, which is destroyed by approximately ten minutes of boiling. For this reason green vegetables, which contain large amounts of the vitamin, should usually be only lightly cooked. Some types like parsley, broccoli and watercress contain far more vitamin C than the citrus fruits. Grains, beans, root vegetables and other foods can be cooked any reasonable length of time without their vitamin content being detrimentally affected.

It is also frequently said that cooking will kill food, and destroy its life force. This life force is actually a dynamic interaction of yin and yang, the forces of heaven and earth. With a knowledge of the yin and yang qualities of foods and cooking techniques this dynamic interaction can be increased to give us a greater charge of energy in our food, rather than diminishing it. When we eat only uncooked foods we are subservient to our environment and the foods available in it. The knowledge of cooking using yin and yang gives us the ability to adapt to different environments and activities, it gives the freedom to freely control our condition and destiny.

Various types of heat have been used in cooking at different times in history. Wood and charcoal have been used for millennia, and more recently coal, gas and electricity have come into use. In the past decade microwaves have become increasingly popular. To understand the effects of these different types of heat they can be arranged on a scale from yang to yin as follows:

wood - charcoal - coal - gas - electricity - microwave

Any of the more yang types of heat from wood to gas can be used to produce a healthy balance in the body. Electric cooking over a long period of time will create an overly yin and weak condition. It is particularly advisable for people suffering from illnesses to use a more yang type of heat than electricity to give them strength to aid their recovery. The use of microwave cooking creates an even more yin condition, and should be avoided by everyone.

Different methods of cooking will change the quality of food in a variety of ways, depending on the yin and yang elements used. The use of heat, salt, and pressure will make food more yang, and adding water will make it more yin. The greater the quantity or the longer the time these elements are applied, the greater will be their effect. With this knowledge different cooking methods can be arranged from yang to yin as follows:

baking - pressure cooking - sauteing - steaming - boiling - pickling - pressing salads - salads

In planning a balanced diet the more balanced cooking methods can be used more often, and the more strongly yin and yang methods less often. Pressure cooking, sauteing, boiling and steaming can all be used more frequently, and baked, pickled, pressed and raw salads used in smaller quantities or less often. It is frequently useful to pressure cook grains like short and medium grain rice, wheat and barley, as these provide the more yang quality needed in the diet, and are given more strength by cooking in this yang manner. As vegetables provide a more yin quality in the diet it is preferable to prepare them with more yin cooking methods most of the time, such as boiling, steaming, pickling and as pressed and raw salads. Some of the beans which require long cooking, such as chickpeas and soya beans, can also be prepared by pressure cooking.

When cooking using the principles of yin and yang, every dish is consciously created with definite qualities, to produce a meal that contains a variety of more yin and more yang qualities that together form a harmonious balance. To achieve this most dishes should be kept simple, with relatively few ingredients and seasonings, and with the minimum amount of interference through over frequent stirring or mixing. If many ingredients and seasonings are combined in one dish without discretion you will receive a confusion of many different energies in it. It can be tempting to throw a lot of different ingredients into a dish to make sure that it is attractive and flavoursome, but as your cooking improves you will be able to produce the most appetising dishes by combining only a few well chosen ingredients in a well prepared manner.

The Importance of Variety

So far in this book we have looked at how to create a balance between more yin and more yang foods. However within this more balanced diet it is important to have plenty of variety. Life is created and sustained by a dynamic interaction of the yin and yang forces. We are alive while the two forces continue to charge our being, and when the charge stops, life stops. The greater the charge of yin and yang forces we receive, the more alive we are, with more energy in our physical, mental and spiritual activities.

The amount of yin and yang charge we receive can be increased through being physically and mentally active. It can also be increased by eating a diet with a strong polarity between more yang and more yin foods and dishes. This can be achieved by making full use of the large number of different types of grains, vegetables, beans, seeds, nuts and fruits, and of different cooking methods and recipes over days and weeks.

Within each meal there should also be a strong polarity

between yin and yang, with some more yang dishes and other more yin dishes. This will occur naturally to some extent with grains, seeds, the smaller beans and root vegetables being more yang, and leafy and other lightly cooked vegetables, nuts and fruits being more yin. The polarity can be further increased through the conscious selection of more yin and yang types of foods and methods of cooking.

When a meal contains variety and polarity it will leave you feeling uplifted and more alive, with a big appetite for getting on with the other activities in your life. If a meal lacks polarity and vitality, then you will also, and you may feel listless and devitalised. Some general ways of increasing the polarity of a meal are described in the following paragraphs.

As the grain is the largest part of the meal, you can begin by choosing which one you will use. If it is a more yang grain, such as millet or buckwheat, a polarity is obtained by preparing vegetable dishes that are more yin, for example by using a greater proportion of leafy types and shorter cooking styles. If the grain is a more yin type, such as barley or corn, then the vegetable dishes can be more yang, with a higher proportion of root varieties and some longer cooking styles.

In the whole meal there should be a variety of cooking methods. If the grain portion of the meal is pressure cooked or baked, the other dishes should be prepared using more yin methods like boiling, steaming or as pressed or raw salad. If the grain is boiled, then some vegetables could be cooked by a more yang method like baking or pressure cooking. There should also be variation in the length of cooking, with some long cooked dishes and other short cooked dishes.

Within the vegetable portion of the meal polarity is produced by including root, round and leafy varieties. When several different vegetable dishes are prepared, some can be cooked longer and others shorter, for example with carrots and swede in a stew and some greens lightly boiled or steamed. If one dish contains a number of vegetables, for example a saute, then all three categories can be included, such as carrot, onion and leek. A few pickles like sauerkraut or brine pickled vegetables can also be eaten with a meal to introduce a very different quality.

We need all of the five main tastes in our food - bitter, salty, sweet, sour and pungent. As the sweet taste is the most balanced we need more of this taste, and smaller amounts of the others. The sweet taste is the natural sweetness of some grains and beans, certain vegetables like onions and carrots, and fruits, and not of the artificial sweetness of sugar or chemical sweeteners. The sour taste can be produced with naturally fermented pickles, including sauerkraut, and good quality vinegars such as rice vinegar. The pungent taste can be given by vegetables with a hot flavour, for example radishes, watercress, spring onions and root ginger. The salty taste can be from seasonings like seasalt, miso and shoyu, and from condiments like gomasio (sesame salt). The bitter taste is often present in vegetables such as lettuce, kale, celery and spring greens. All or most of these tastes should be present in the main meal of the day, or at least eaten in the course of one day.

When a meal is both balanced and contains variety, it will look appetising, with many different colours and textures, and will leave you feeling completely satisfied. If you feel the urge to look for additional "nibbles" after the meal, it must either have been imbalanced or lacking in some basic quality. If the meal was overall too yang you will be attracted to sweet tasting foods and other yin items. If it was too yin you will be attracted to salty foods and other yang items. If every dish was wet, you will seek something dry, and too dry a meal will leave you seeking something wet or succulent. If a certain taste was missing from the meal you may then go hunting for it in some readily available form, for example if there was no sweet taste you may want some dried fruits or barley malt.

These after meal cravings provide a good chance to learn how to prepare better meals. You can work out what quality you are looking for using your knowledge of the yin and yang nature of foods and the five tastes. This quality was missing from the meal, so you can think about possible dishes with this quality that you could have included in the meal. Cooking meals that are balanced and contain all the qualities necessary for our health needs an understanding of yin and yang, experimentation, and creativity. This makes cooking a great art of endless interest and learning, a far more enjoyable pass time than just producing sensorially satisfying food. As with learning any art it is useful to study other people's work, so it is very useful to follow some cooking classes or to share other people's meals in developing your own cooking.

Planning a Day's Meals

Once the principles of the balanced diet have been appreciated, the next concern is how to put it into practice. The first step is to plan your day's meals, after which you can look in detail at how to prepare individual recipes. (Various cookery books containing recipes and meal plans can be found in Further Reading). Changing your diet can seem a big hurdle, but with proper planning it becomes a much simpler process. In this section some guidelines and suggestions are made for what you can plan for each meal of the day.

Because of the time taken to prepare whole foods it is a good idea to spend a longer time preparing the main meal of the day, which for most people is the evening meal, and make the others quickly prepared meals. By cooking larger quantities of dishes at the main meal, some can be kept for the other meals to save having to start from scratch in their preparation. This is particularly true for grains and beans, which need a longer cooking time.

To obtain the maximum amount of energy over the day we can plan our eating according to the daily cycle of energy. The night, being colder and darker, is a more yin time, and the day, being warmer and lighter, is more yang. As with the dietary adjustments for different climates and seasons, we can harmonise with these daily changes in our environment by making ourselves of the opposite and complimentary nature.

This can be achieved by eating more yin food during the yang day, and more yang food during the yin night. Practically, breakfast and lunch are eaten during the day, and so should be lighter meals, and supper is eaten at the beginning of the night, and so should be more yang.

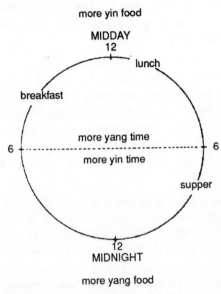

Fig. 8. Harmonizing meals with the daily cycle of energy.

For breakfast, grains can provide a long lasting source of energy for the morning. These can be prepared softer than usual as a porridge to form a lighter or more yin dish. This can be made by cooking whole grains like barley, rice, millet or oats for a longer time and with more water than usual. A quicker porridge can be made by cooking the grain from yesterday's main meal with more water, and sometimes by using rolled oats or barley. They can occasionally be made from a sugar free soya milk if you want a creamier texture, and garnished with sesame salt or roasted seeds. To be digestible grains need to be cooked with water, so the raw grains of muesli, and the dry roasted grains of 'granola' and similar preparations, will tax the digestive system. They often cause fermentation and gas production, and will not provide us with so much energy.

Other possible breakfasts include a lightly seasoned soup made with vegetables or vegetables combined with yesterday's grains, mashed tofu scrambled in a frying pan with shoyu and chopped spring onions or parsley, or if you want something lighter some wholewheat or udon noodles in a vegetable soup or with steamed vegetables.

Lunch can be mainly made up of a selection of the grain, vegetable and bean dishes cooked for the previous day's main meal, bearing in mind that this should be a lighter meal. If you eat lunch away from home, these can be taken in a suitable container, together with soup or tea in a thermos flask. If you are at home you could also eat these foods, or prepare a quick meal such as noodles, either in a soup or with some quickly prepared vegetables.

On most days of the week the main meal of the day, which is usually supper, should be a complete and well balanced meal that contains the full variety of foods in the diet. It should include a soup if one has not already been eaten that day, a whole cereal grain, a variety of root, round and green vegetables, and a dish higher in protein such as beans, tofu or fish. Several times a week a separate dish made with a seaweed can also be eaten. Various pickles are a good addition and can be eaten at most meals. The meal could be followed by a dessert with fruits, grain sweeteners, or other ingredients, but this is not essential at every meal. Your main meal may look something like this:-

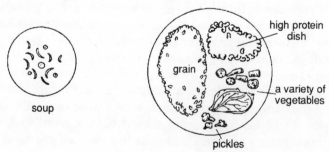

soup

grain

high protein dish

a variety of vegetables

pickles

The different food groups are shown separately, but they could sometimes be combined, for example the high protein food could be in the form of bean soup, or the grains and vegetables could be in a stew.

Besides eating two or three meals a day, you may sometimes want some between meal snacks. For this you could use rice cakes (made with puffed rice grains), some roasted pumpkin or sunflower seeds, or roasted nuts. If you are at home you could of course also eat a little of any grain and vegetable dishes left over from previous meals.

Imbalance Equals Disease

Being truly healthy does not just mean not having any obvious symptoms or illness. Many people in this condition suddenly develop a serious and sometimes fatal illness, such as cancer, a heart attack, or a stroke. Obviously their condition must have been degenerating over a long period to suddenly suffer such a serious illness. Rather, health is a constant process of maintaining an internal balance, preventing sickness not only in the present, but also in the future. All illness is the exception to the healthy state that it is possible for us to enjoy, produced by our lack of knowledge of nature's laws. Even with infectious diseases, we will only be susceptible to invasion by bacteria or viruses if the body's internal condition is weak. A healthy diet combined with activity can build up strong defences to infections.

The prevalent diet in Western countries is primarily made up of the extreme yin and extreme yang foods, with little of the more balanced cereal grains, vegetables and beans. Consequently people suffer from a multitude of physical and mental illnesses caused by an imbalance in their condition.

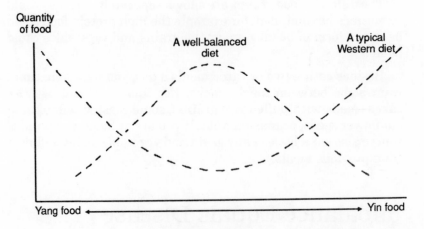

Fig. 9. A typical Western diet and a well-balanced diet.

All sicknesses fall into one of three categories, those of a yang nature, those of a yin nature, and those with a nature produced by a combination of yin and yang. Understanding the cause of sicknesses in this way leads to a simple understanding of how they may be improved or cured. Some examples will make this clear.

If excessive amounts of yin foods are eaten, such as sugar, spices, highly processed and chemicalised foods, or tropical fruits and vegetables, various ailments involving the expansion and weakening of organs and systems will arise. The intestines will become loose and expanded, causing either chronic diarrhoea or constipation, the development of diverticula, and later colitis or enteritis. Other organs will become inflamed, such as the tonsils, adenoids, lymph glands, and the lining of the upper stomach leading to the formation of ulcers in this region. Expansion of the cells and blood vessels of the brain brings on certain forms of headaches and migraines, which in many peoples experience are brought on by wine, chocolate or sugar - all very yin items. Meningitis, asthma, hayfever and bronchitis, cystitis and hernias are also caused by the expansion and weakening of various organs and structures.

An excess of yin foods also leads to psychological imbalance. Hallucinatory drugs are well known to 'expand the consciousness', a phrase that accurately describes the effects of these extremely yin chemicals. At the same time their frequent use also produces difficulties in maintaining concentration, and in dealing with every day practical concerns. All the more extreme yin foods have the same kind of effects to a lesser extent, especially alcohol and sugar. It is interesting to note that these very yin foods often become addictive - drugs are seen as a serious problem, but alcoholism is more widespread, and the great majority of people in Western countries are addicted to sugar. (If you regularly eat sugar, try cutting it out of your diet for a week, and see how you feel. Remember to also stop eating other foods high in simple sugars, for example honey, molasses, jams and many sauces.)

Other effects of the over-consumption of yin foods are excessive worry and fearfulness, over-excitability and emotionality, nervousness, and in the extreme, schizophrenia. Recent reports by the McCarrison Society and researchers in hospitals, prisons and American adolescent detention centres have shown that sugar greatly increases hyperactivity and violent behaviour. Sugar is undoubtedly the cause of many problems for individuals and in society.

These more yin conditions will be improved by avoiding extreme yin foods, and eating the more balanced diet described in previous sections of this book. The effectiveness of the diet will be improved by selecting the more yang varieties within each food group - among the grains short grain brown rice and millet, among beans aduki beans, green or brown lentils and chickpeas, and with vegetables more roots. Seaweeds like kelp, hiziki and arame are also very beneficial due to their high mineral content. More longer cooking methods, with the use of a little more salt, can also be used.

When a person consumes a greater proportion of yang foods, especially eggs, red meat, cheese and excessive amounts of salt, various parts of the body become hardened and constricted. This impairs their normal functioning and leads to sickness. The excess of saturated animal fat from these foods is well known to be a cause of arteriosclerosis in which the arteries become coated in fatty material, mainly cholesterol, with subsequent thickening and hardening of the artery walls. The blood flow through the arteries is restricted and can give rise to angina or a heart attack. The excessive use of salt has been shown to contract the many small arteries in the body, restricting the flow of blood and causing high blood pressure.

Other illnesses caused by an overly yang condition includes some diseases involving the stiffening of joints such as gout and lockjaw, most cases of menstrual cramps, and mental imbalances characterised by deep tension, hardening and stiffness. This includes stubbornness, inflexibility, narrow thinking, deep-seated tension, and frequent anger and irritability. In the extreme the over-consumption of yang foods causes severe disturbances, including paranoia.

These conditions will be improved by avoiding extreme yang foods, and eating the balanced diet. In these cases the diet can have a more yin emphasis with less fish and more fruits. Within each food group the more yin types can be eaten more often, for example among grains barley and corn, and with vegetables more leafy greens. Lighter cooking styles can be used, possibly including more salads, with less salt and salty seasonings like miso and shoyu.

Some illnesses arise from a combination of both extreme yin and extreme yang foods. This includes many skin ailments such as eczema and psoriasis, the formation of gall bladder and kidney stones, and of breast cysts and cataracts. A diet containing both extremes of yin and yang foods also produces emotional instability, with frequent changes between opposite emotions. There will be a mixture of those emotions and attitudes caused by eating a predominantly yin and predominantly yang diet described above.

With illness of this category improvement will follow avoiding all extreme yin and extreme yang foods, and eating the balanced diet. Within the balanced diet the more extreme foods should be minimised, such as fish and fruits. In each food group more of the centrally balanced foods can be eaten, for example among grains, short grain brown rice, wheat and barley. The use of salt and salty seasonings should be moderate. In cooking the most yang methods like baking and the most yin methods like pressed salads and raw foods should not be used.

This approach to understanding disease considers the overall condition of a person, and not just their symptoms. The advice based on this understanding can not only help improve a particular health problem, but will also bring the whole person back into balance, with many benefits physically, emotionally and mentally.

This section is intended to give a simple introduction to understanding the cause of disease, and how it may be improved, using yin and yang. With a deeper understanding of yin and yang applied to food, the structure and functioning of the body and oriental diagnosis, more detailed dietary advice can be used to correct internal imbalances in particular organs and systems within the body. If you wish to use diet to cure a specific illness it is advisable to receive individual dietary guidance for your own unique condition from a qualified counsellor experienced in using the theory of yin and yang to promote health. Addresses of such people are given at the back of this book.

The Benefits of Balance

When we make balance in our daily food we create a balance between opposite chemicals and functions in our body. This includes the sodium/potassium and acid/alkali balance of the blood and body cells, the secretion of hormones with opposing effects, the sympathetic and parasympathetic branches of the autonomic nervous system, and the left and right and inner and outer regions of the brain. This produces harmony throughout our being, in our physical, psychological and spiritual existence.

Eating the balanced diet will also result in the body discharging or eliminating various foods and toxins previously eaten in excess of the body's needs. Everyone who has eaten a typical Western diet has these excessive substances stored and accumulated in the body, which can include animal fats, vegetable oils, the products of sugar metabolism, chemicals, drugs, and other toxins. If the balanced diet is eaten in the correct proportions it will provide all our nutritional requirements while avoiding these various excesses. When the body is no longer forced to consume them, it will naturally begin to discharge the stored materials.

As an internal balance is restored and past excesses are discharged, many varied benefits are experienced. Some of the more commonly found effects are described here.

The physical benefits of a balanced diet include an increase in energy and vitality, which allow one to participate in and enjoy life more fully. One's sleep tends to get deeper and more restful, while at the same time becoming shorter. Many minor ailments and problems recede, and body weight tends to come to its natural level. Furthermore, when the application of a balanced diet is combined with a basic knowledge of oriental diagnosis and yin and yang applied to the physiology of the body it is possible to avoid suffering from the degenerative illnesses that affect nearly every individual and family in the modern world. This includes arteriosclerosis, heart disease and failure, stroke, cancer, arthritis and rheumatism, kidney and gall bladder stones, hypoglycaemia and diabetes, glaucoma, cataracts, senile dementia, and many others.

Our physical condition and psychological and spiritual state are not separate, as they are often considered to be in Western thought, but are different aspects of one whole. Therefore establishing balanced and harmonious bodily functioning is the foundation for emotional, mental and spiritual health and happiness. A few examples will illustrate this connection.

It is undeniable that when we are suffering from a physical illness we also feel emotionally and mentally depleted. Even when we do not have a specific illness our body may be functioning far below its possible level of efficiency. As the health improves and one's energy increases, depression and negativity will be replaced with a positive and optimistic attitude to life.

Stress is the result of a lack of energy and adaptability in dealing with the demands and challenges of daily life. The basic cause of this condition is usually a lack of energy and flexibility in the body. With improved health, the ability to quickly adapt and act appropriately in changing situations increases, and many situations that were previously found stressful can be coped with with ease.

Achieving balance in the physical body produces greater emotional and psychological equilibrium. With an overly yin or yang condition one is trapped in certain emotions and attitudes, which can be difficult to get out of solely through conscious effort or by using techniques for psychological release or change. As one becomes biologically balanced, it becomes much easier to become free of old habitual ways of thinking and reacting. When one becomes overall more yang, one can be obsessed by order, discipline, and tidiness, with a more dominating and insensitive attitude. Often deep tension is a chronic problem, and is accompanied by a need to always be busy and working, with difficulties in ever stopping and relaxing. When one becomes overall more yin, one can be trapped in a lack of self-confidence and self-respect, with excessive worry, fear, self-pity or over-sensitivity. Problems can be experienced in being down to earth, practical and realistic, with difficulties in ordering one's life, fulfilling basic needs and upholding commitments.

Restoring a balance within the body makes it easier to lose these delusional states and difficulties. One can develop inner peace, inward confidence and outward humbleness, and a new ability to deal with everyday living. You can become free to choose when to be organised, busy and efficient, and when to be relaxed, enjoying company and pleasurable pursuits.

As various physical, emotional and mental changes take place, the ability to maintain and enjoy relationships with other people can increase. When physical and psychological problems are replaced by a healthy and balanced disposition, more energy and concern can be turned outwards from oneself to other people. To build and maintain satisfying relationships with parents, children, friends and partners it is necessary to develop a balance between more yin and more yang qualities. More yin qualities include sensitivity, the ability to be receptive and listening, patience and compassion. Yang qualities include dependability and constancy, resourcefulness, and the ability to provide steady support. The balance produced at different levels of oneself by following the balanced diet allows these opposite qualities to develop in harmony with each other in relationships.

One of the biggest sources of unhappiness in many people today is a spiritual poorness, manifesting as a lack of direction and purpose in life. Often we take on the generally excepted roles and attitudes of our society or a particular group, rather than discovering our real potentials, feelings and thoughts. A more balanced condition can give us greater mental peace and clarity, and the unfolding of our intuition, producing a clearer view of oneself and one's life. Mental dilemmas and confusions can disappear, and the personally important aspects of life become more obvious. One can gain more motivation and direction, a greater sense of purpose and fulfilment. It gives the chance to fully realise the enormous potentials that each of us has been given in this lifetime.

As we refine our understanding of yin and yang and its application to following a balanced diet, its benefits unfold over time, becoming more profound over days, months and years. The harmony it creates progresses to deeper levels of ourselves, and as different parts come into balance various impediments to our happiness give way to a new and positive way of life.

Menu Plans

In this section there are menu plans for two full week's meals. Recipes for all these dishes will be found in the next section.

From these menu plans you can learn how to create balance in your cooking, in individual meals, over one day, and with the seasons. You may need to make adjustments in your diet to suit your personal condition; if you have become overall too yang, then you can use more yin ingredients and cooking methods as in the summer menu plans. If you have become too yin then you can use more of the more yang ingredients and cooking styles of the winter menus.

The plans are also designed to show you the wide variety of possibilities for dishes at different meals. You may find that certain dishes suit your appetite and life style better, for example breakfast can consist of a soup, or porridge with vegetables; lunch can be made up of the dishes of yesterday's main meal, can be a freshly cooked meal, or a combination of the two; supper usually includes soup, whole grains, beans or fish, a variety of vegetables, and sometimes a seaweed, but within this basic plan there are many ways of preparing each type of food.

It is important to find the particular dishes that you and your family and friends like best, however do not fall into a set pattern of cooking a small fixed number or recipes, as this will create boredom with the food and a stagnation of energy in the body. Always be expanding your scope of recipes, and once the basic principles of cooking by yin and yang have been grasped, experiment yourself with new recipes and combinations of ingredients.

Summer Menus

BREAKFAST   **LUNCH**

Monday

- Soft Rice.
- Steamed spring cabbage.

- Wholewheat or udon noodles.
- Onion, broccoli and green beans sauted with water.
- Brine pickles.

Tuesday

- Rolled oat porridge.
- Boiled broccoli.

- Fried rice using yesterday's rice, with onion, mushrooms, beansprouts and spring onions.
- Sauerkraut.

Wednesday

- Whole oat porridge.
- Brine pickles.

- Rice and wheat from yesterday.
- Steamed carrot and courgette.
- Blanched watercress.

Thursday

- Miso soup from yesterday.

- Sourdough bread.
- Salad of grated carrot and cabbage with tahini dressing.

SUPPER

- Quick miso soup.
- Boiled short grain rice.
- Aduki beans cooked with kombu, carrot and onion.
- Arame and toasted sesame seeds.
- Pressed salad of lettuce and cucumber with tofu dressing.

- Corn and Chinese cabbage miso soup.
- Pressure-cooked short grain rice and wheat.
- Waterless style carrots and kombu.
- Chickpea pate.
- Cucumber and wakame salad with rice vinegar.
- Strawberry jelly.

- Pearl barley and onion miso soup.
- Boiled medium grain rice.
- Boiled carrot, onion, and tofu with kuzu gravy made from the cooking water.
- Blanched spring cabbage cut finely and mixed with sauerkraut.

- Pressure-cooked short grain rice and barley.
- Lentils cooked with wakame and spring onions.
- Steamed daikon (mouli).
- Blanched salad of cauliflower, celery and watercress with rice vinegar and shoyu dressing.
- Slices of fresh melon.

BREAKFAST	**LUNCH**

Friday

- Rolled oat porridge.
- Scrambled tofu with spring onions.

- Rice and barley from yesterday.
- Lentils from yesterday.
- Blanched salad from yesterday.

Saturday

- Soft Millet and onion using yesterday's grain.
- Brine pickles.

- Corn on the cob.
- Hiziki salad from yesterday.

Sunday

- Soft rice made from yesterday's grain.
- Blanched salad of cabbage.

- Rice from yesterday mixed with roasted pumpkin seeds.
- Boiled cauliflower, broccoli and runner beans.

SUPPER

- Cauliflower and onion miso soup.
- Millet and onion croquettes.
- Sauted carrot mixed with roasted sesame seeds.
- Hiziki salad with tofu dressing.

- Shoyu broth with carrot matchsticks, onions, mushrooms, tofu and spring onions.
- Boiled medium grain rice.
- Shallow boiled plaice with shoyu, ginger juice and rice vinegar.
- Salad of chopped lettuce, cucumber, radishes and mustard cress with umeboshi dressing.
- Lightly stewed fresh apples with soya milk custard.

- Onion and wakame miso soup.
- Pressure-cooked short grain rice mixed with blanched peas, green beans and roasted sunflower seeds.
- Waterless style carrot, turnip and kombu.
- Chickpea salad with onion, celery, radish and lettuce.

Winter Menus

BREAKFAST	**LUNCH**

Monday

- Soft rice.
- Boiled leeks.

- Wholewheat, udon or buckwheat noodles in shoyu broth.

Tuesday

- Whole oat porridge.
- Steamed watercress.

- Rice from yesterday.
- Aduki beans from yesterday.
- Blanched salad of cauliflower and brussel sprouts.

Wednesday

- Rolled oat porridge.
- Boiled cabbage.

- Millet and onion from yesterday.
- Quick saute of carrot, onion and leek.

Thursday

- Soft millet cooked with onion and mushrooms.

- Rice and chestnuts from yesterday.
- Steamed broccoli.

SUPPER

- Daikon and wakame miso soup.
- Pressure-cooked short grain rice.
- Aduki beans cooked with kombu and carrots.
- Arame and onions.
- Pressed salad of finely cut cabbage with rice vinegar.
- Pear and apple crumble.

- Lentil soup with onion and parsley.
- Millet and onion.
- Waterless style carrot, burdock and kombu.
- Boiled kale.

- Shoyu broth with onion, tofu and parsley.
- Pressure-cooked short grain rice and chestnuts.
- Baked parsnips.
- Hiziki mixed with roasted and sliced almonds.
- Blanched salad of cauliflower, cauliflower greens and spring onions with tofu dressing.
- Oatmeal raisin cookies.

- Aduki bean soup.
- Pressure-cooked short grain rice and barley.
- Long saute of carrot, swede and brussel sprouts.
- Boiled leeks mixed with umeboshi dressing.

BREAKFAST

LUNCH

Friday

- Soft rice made from yesterday's grain cooked with onion and swede.
- Brine pickles.

- Fried whole wheat spaghetti, udon or buckwheat noodles with onion, leek and tofu.

Saturday

- Miso soup from yesterday with sourdough bread.

- Rice from yesterday.
- Boiled carrot, turnip and turnip greens.

Sunday

- Rolled oat porridge.

- Steamed leeks.

- Barley and lentil stew from yesterday.
- Sauerkraut.

SUPPER

- Onion and wakame miso soup.
- Boiled short grain rice.
- Baked cod with shoyu, mustard and rice vinegar.
- Kombu and carrot rolls.
- Steamed kale and cauliflower cut finely and mixed with sauerkraut.
- Baked apples with soya milk custard.

- Barley and lentil stew with carrots, onions and brussel sprouts.
- Blanched salad of Chinese cabbage with rice vinegar and shoyu dressing.

- Quick miso soup.
- Pressure-cooked short grain rice and aduki beans.
- Waterless style parsnip, swede, brussel sprouts and kombu.
- Quick saute of mushrooms, tofu, beansprouts and watercress.

Recipes

In this section there is a selection of recipes which you can use in preparing the meals given in the menu plans, or in planning your own meals. Once these have been mastered you are recommended to consult some of the cookery books given in Further Reading to extend your range of dishes.

Grains

Pressure Cooked Brown Rice

1 cup short or medium grain rice
1¼-1½ cups water
1 pinch sea salt

Place the rice in a stainless steel pressure cooker, add water to cover and gently stir with your hand to wash it, then pour off the dirty water. Repeat once or twice, or until the washing water is clear. Add the required amount of water and salt, cover, and bring up to pressure. When the pressure is up turn the heat very low. A flame deflector can also be placed under the pot to prevent burning. Cook for 45-50 minutes.

At the end of cooking turn the heat off and allow the pressure to drop slowly. After 5 minutes the pressure can be allowed to escape by putting a spoon handle under the pressure valve. Take the rice out one spoonful at a time and spread in a serving bowl, carefully separating the individual grains before removing the next spoonful. This rice will have a delicious nutty flavour.

Variations: Sometimes roasted seeds or nuts can be mixed with the cooked rice, for example sunflower seeds or almonds. To cook larger amounts simply use the same proportions of water and salt to a larger quantity of rice.

54

Boiled Rice

1 cup short or medium grain rice
2 cups water
1 pinch sea salt

Place the rice in a saucepan and wash as for pressure cooked rice. Add the water and salt, cover with a lid, and bring to the boil. Turn the heat very low and simmer for 50-60 minutes or until all the water has been absorbed. Remove the rice as in the above recipe.

Soft Rice

1 cup short or medium grain rice
5 cups water
1 pinch sea salt

Wash the rice and either pressure cook or boil as in the above recipes for 1-1½ hours.

The rice becomes very creamy and makes an excellent breakfast porridge. Soft rice can also be made with cooked rice from the day before by adding 3 cups of water per cup of rice and cooking for 30-35 minutes.

Variations: soft rice can be cooked with vegetables, such as carrot and onion or Chinese cabbage.

Rice with other Grains

1 cup short or medium grain rice
¼ cup of one of pot or pearl barley, wheat, millet or oats
1½ - 1¾ cups water
1 pinch sea salt

These combinations can be cooked in the same way as pressure cooked rice, by placing the grains together in the pot. However barley, wheat and oats take longer to cook than rice, so they should be soaked for 2-3 hours before adding to the rice.

These make nice variations to plain rice.

Rice with Beans or Dried Chestnuts

1 cup short or medium grain rice
⅛ cup aduki or black soya beans or dried chestnuts
1¾-2 cups water
2 pinches sea salt

Spread the beans on a flat plate and pick out any stones or impurities. Place the beans or chestnuts in a pressure cooker and wash as described above for rice. As beans and dried chestnuts need longer cooking than rice, boil with the water for 30-40 minutes by themselves. Wash the rice separately, then add to the beans or chestnuts with the salt and pressure cook for 45-50 minutes. Serve as with plain rice.

Fried Rice

2 cups cooked rice
1-2 teaspoons sesame oil
1 medium onion sliced finely
1 medium carrot sliced finely or cut into matchsticks
¼ lb. mushrooms sliced finely
1 cup beansprouts
1 teaspoon shoyu

Brush a frying pan with the oil and heat for a minute. Spread the onion in the pan, then the other vegetables, and the rice on top. Cover the pan and cook on a low flame for 10 minutes. Add the shoyu and cook another 5 minutes. There should be no need to stir during cooking, just mix together before serving.

Variations: use other combinations of vegetables. Tofu can also be added to make a more complete meal.

Millet

1 cup millet
2½ cups boiling water
1 pinch sea salt

Wash the millet in the same way as rice, or in a sieve under a tap. Lightly roast in a dry frying pan on a medium heat for 5 minutes until slightly golden. Stir occasionally to prevent burning. Roasting gives millet a beautifully nutty flavour. Add the millet and salt to the boiling water, bring back to the boil, cover and turn heat to low. Simmer for 30-35 minutes or until all the water has been absorbed. Gently remove a spoonful at a time into a serving bowl.

Variations: saute ½lb onions in a little sesame oil until golden and place in the boiling water before the millet. While the millet is still warm it can be shaped in the hands to form burgers or croquettes. Burgers can be fried in a little oil, and are particularly enjoyed by children.

Soft Millet

1 cup millet
4-5 cups water
1 pinch sea salt

Wash, roast and cook as in the above recipe for 45 minutes or until soft. Soft millet can be used as a breakfast cereal.

Whole Oat Porridge

1 cup whole oats
5-6 cups water
1 pinch sea salt

Wash the oats as with rice and place in a saucepan with the water and salt. Cover and bring to the boil. Reduce the heat to very low and simmer for several hours, or overnight in the winter. Alternatively cook for ¾ hour the night before, and another ½ hour in the morning.

This traditional Scottish recipe is extremely creamy and very warming on winter mornings.

Rolled Oat Porridge

1 cup rolled oats
2½-3 cups water
1 pinch sea salt

It is preferable to use medium rolled or jumbo oats as they have been milled less, and have a fuller flavour. Place the oats, water and salt in a saucepan, bring to the boil and reduce heat to low. Simmer for 10-30 minutes, depending on the size of the flakes. Garnish with gomasio (sesame salt) or roasted seeds.

Variations: this porridge could occasionally be cooked with sugar free soya milk for a creamier taste. Barley malt could be added if you want a sweeter taste.

Barley and Lentil Stew

1 cup barley
3-4 cups water
¼ cup lentils
1 onion diced
1 cup carrots diced
1 cup brussel sprouts
3 celery stalks diced
½ cup button mushrooms
½ teaspoon sea salt

Wash the barley and lentils individually in a sieve under a tap, place all the ingredients in a saucepan, cover and bring to the boil. Reduce heat to low and simmer for 1½ hours. For a more warming dish in the winter, once the stew boils, put it in a casserole with the lid on in the oven at 250F (gas mark ½) for 1½-2 hours.

Corn on the Cob

Steam or boil whole fresh cobs for 10 minutes or until soft. These are delicious as a light grain when they are in season in the summer.

Noodles and Broth

1 packet buckwheat or udon noodles, or wholewheat spaghetti
2 pints water
3 inch piece kombu seaweed
3-4 fresh or dried (shitake) mushrooms sliced
2-3 tablespoons shoyu

Boil 2-3 pints of water, add noodles and simmer for 10-15 minutes. You can check when they are done by breaking a piece, when the inside and outside are the same colour they are done. Remove noodles from saucepan into a sieve and rinse under a tap to stop them sticking together.

Start making the broth once the noodles have come to the boil. Wipe the kombu with a damp cloth to remove excess salt and place in a saucepan with the water and mushrooms (dried mushrooms must first be soaked for 15 minutes and their stems removed). Bring to the boil, reduce the heat and simmer for 5 minutes. Remove the kombu, and keep for another recipe. Add the shoyu and simmer 5 minutes more. Place noodles in broth to warm up, then serve. Garnish with chopped spring onions, chives or toasted nori seaweed cut into 1 inch squares.

Variations: use other vegetables, e.g. finely sliced carrot and watercress. Small cubes of tofu can also be added.

Fried Noodles and Vegetables

1 packet buckwheat or udon noodles, or wholewheat spaghetti
1 tablespoon sesame oil
1 medium onion finely sliced
1 cup cabbage finely sliced
½ cup mushrooms finely sliced
½ cup chopped spring onions
1 tablespoon shoyu

Cook the noodles as in the previous recipe, rinse and drain. Brush a frying pan with the oil, spread out the onion, cabbage and mushrooms, and the noodles on top. Cover and cook on a low flame for 4-5 minutes. Mix noodles and vegetables, add shoyu and cook for 3 minutes. Add spring onions and serve.

Variations: onion, beansprouts, watercress and tofu.

Sourdough Bread

3lb. wholewheat flour
2 tablespoons sesame oil (optional)
¼-½ teaspoon sea salt

Make a starter by mixing ½ cup of flour with enough water to make a thin batter. Cover with a damp cloth and stand in a warm place for 3-4 days or until it smells sour, but not mouldy.

Mix the remaining flour and salt, then rub in the oil. Add the starter and just enough water to form a thick dough, and knead 200-300 times. Oil 2 bread pans with sesame oil and place in dough. Cover with a damp cloth and let sit in a warm place for 8-12 hours or until it has risen to twice the size. Bake at 300F (gas mark 4) for 1¼-1½ hours.

Sourdough bread can be very sweet and delicious. If making it regularly, remove a little of the kneaded dough and mix with a little water to begin your next starter.

Soups

Vegetable Miso Soup

½ cup onions thinly sliced
3-4 inch piece of wakame seaweed
1 pint water
½ tablespoon miso

Quickly rinse wakame in water to remove excess salt and soak in ½ cup of water for 5 minutes, then slice into ½ inch pieces. Place wakame with its soaking water and onions in a saucepan and add rest of water. Bring to the boil, cover, and simmer 10-15 minutes or until tender. Reduce flame to very low so there is no bubbling. Puree the miso with ½ cup of the soup and return to the soup. Allow to cook 3-4 minutes without bubbling to preserve beneficial enzymes in the miso, and serve. Garnish with chopped parsley, spring onions or watercress, or grated root ginger.

The soup should not taste too salty or too bland. A little more miso will be needed in the winter, and a little less in the summer. Barley miso is the most balanced and the best to use regularly, hatcho (100% soya bean) and brown rice can be used occasionally. Hatcho miso is more yang and can be used more often in the winter; brown rice miso is more yin and can be used more often in the summer.

Variations: cauliflower and onion, wakame and daikon (mouli); corn cut from a cob and Chinese cabbage.

Quick Miso Soup

⅓ cup chopped spring onions
1 pint water
1 sheet nori seaweed cut into 1 inch squares
½-1 tablespoon miso

Boil the water, reduce the flame to very low so there is no bubbling. Remove ¼ cup and puree the miso in it, and return to the pan. Add the spring onions and cook 3-4 minutes. Add nori and serve.

Shoyu Broth

3 inch piece of kombu seaweed
3-4 fresh or dried (shitake) mushrooms sliced
½ cup tofu sliced
¼ cup chopped spring onions
1 pint water
1-2 tablespoons shoyu

If you are using dried mushrooms soak them for 10 minutes and cut off the stalks. Wipe the kombu with a damp cloth to remove excess salt and place with the water in a pot. Simmer for 5 minutes (this adds minerals and much flavour). Remove kombu and use in another recipe. Add mushrooms and tofu, simmer for 5-10 minutes. Add shoyu, simmer 2-3 minutes more. Add spring onions and serve.

Variations: onion, tofu and watercress; Chinese cabbage and chives; sauteed onion and parsley.

Lentil Soup

1 cup green or brown lentils
2 medium onions diced
1 carrot diced
¼ cup chopped parsley
2 pints water
1 pinch sea salt
½-1 tablespoon shoyu

Wash the lentils in a sieve under a tap. Spread the onion on the bottom of a saucepan, then add the carrot, and the lentils on top. Add the water and a pinch of salt and bring to the boil. Reduce flame to low, cover and simmer 50 minutes. Add parsley and shoyu, simmer 10 minutes more and serve.

Variations: the same recipe can be used to make a creamy split pea soup, using 1 cup of split peas instead of the lentils.

Aduki Bean Soup

1 cup aduki beans
2 inch piece kombu seaweed
2 medium onions sliced
2 medium carrots sliced
2 pints water
½-1 tablespoon shoyu

Wipe excess salt off kombu with a damp cloth, soak for 10-15 minutes and slice into thin strips. Put the beans on a flat plate, pick out stones and impurities, then wash in a sieve under a tap.

Put kombu, beans and water in a saucepan, bring to the boil, cover and reduce heat to low. Simmer for 1 hour. Add onion, carrot and shoyu and simmer ½ hour more. Garnish with chopped spring onions or parsley to serve.

Variations: vary the vegetables, e.g. parsnip and leek, carrot and celery.

Pearl Barley and Onion Soup

½ cup pearl barley
3 medium onions sliced thinly
1 teaspoon sesame oil
2 pints water
1 pinch sea salt
1-2 tablespoons shoyu

Wash the barley, then boil in the water for ¾ hour. Saute the onions in the oil with a pinch of salt until golden brown. Add the onions to the barley and cook another 20 minutes. Add shoyu and cook 10 minutes more. Garnish with chopped parsley or nori seaweed cut into 1 inch squares.

Vegetables

Boiling

Place 1-2 inches of water in a saucepan, add a pinch of salt and bring to the boil. Add vegetables for between 1 and 10 minutes, then remove and serve. Keep remaining water for a soup or other recipe.

Most vegetables can be cooked in this way. Some cook very fast, for example watercress and spring onions, and need only 1-2 minutes. Others like carrots and swede need longer.

Tasty combinations of boiled vegetables include broccoli and cauliflower; carrots, onions and peas; cabbage, corn and tofu; leeks with umeboshi (pickled plums).

Steaming

Place half an inch of water in a saucepan and then a vegetable steamer. Add sliced vegetables and sprinkle with a pinch of sea salt. Cover, bring to the boil, and steam 2-7 minutes. Remove vegetables and serve. Save remaining water for other dishes.

Green vegetables generally take 1-4 minutes steaming, round and root vegetables take a little longer. If you do not have a steamer, put half an inch of water in a pot, add vegetables and salt, cover and steam.

This is an ideal way of cooking greens like kale, spring cabbage, Chinese cabbage, watercress, and turnip tops, and can be used frequently.

Baking

½ lb. carrots, parsnips or Hokkaido pumpkin cut in thick slices
1-2 teaspoons shoyu

Place the vegetables on a baking tray, add ¼-½ inch of water and sprinkle the shoyu over the vegetables. Bake at 400F (gas mark 6) for 40 minutes or until soft. Add more water if necessary.

These vegetables become very sweet cooked in this way.

Quick Saute

½ cup carrot cut into thin matchsticks
½ cup onions sliced thinly
½ cup cabbage sliced thinly
½ cup beansprouts
¼ cup mushrooms sliced thinly
1 teaspoon sesame oil
1-2 pinches sea salt
1-2 teaspoons shoyu
1-2 teaspoons rice vinegar

Brush frying pan with oil and heat for 1 minute. Add the vegetables and sprinkle the salt over them. Cook 5 minutes on a medium flame, gently turning the vegetables occasionally. Add the shoyu and vinegar and cook 1-2 minutes more, then serve. The vegetables should be tender but still crisp.

If you are limiting the amount of oil that you eat, replace the oil with 2-3 tablespoons of water.

Variations: Onion, Chinese cabbage, corn, watercress and tofu; parsnip, onion, celery and broccoli.

Long Saute

½ cup carrot cut in thick matchsticks or slices
½ cup broccoli cut into pieces
½ cup onion cut in thick slices
½ cup cauliflower cut into pieces
1 teaspoon sesame oil
1-2 pinches sea salt
1-2 teaspoons shoyu

Brush pan with oil and heat for 1 minute. Add vegetables, sprinkle the salt over them, and cook on a medium heat for 5 minutes, turning occasionally. Add water to just cover the bottom of the pan. Cover and cook 10-15 minutes, adding more water if necessary to prevent burning. Add shoyu and cook 2-3 minutes more without a cover to allow any remaining water to evaporate.

Variations: parsnip, onion, cabbage and tofu; burdock and carrot; carrot and roasted sesame seeds.

Waterless Style (Nishimi)

6 inch piece of kombu seaweed
1 cup carrot cut into 1-2 inch chunks
1 medium onion cut in quarters
1 cup cabbage cut in 1-2 inch wide slices through the stem
1 pinch séa salt
1-2 teaspoons shoyu

Wipe the kombu with a damp cloth to remove excess salt, soak for 20-30 minutes and cut into 1 inch pieces. Put the kombu in the bottom of a heavy pot that has a tight fitting lid. Add vegetables, ½ inch of water and salt. Cover and bring to the boil, then turn to medium low heat and cook for 15-30 minutes. If necessary add more water to prevent burning. Add shoyu and cook 3 minutes longer. Any juice left can be served with the vegetables, and is very delicious.

This method of cooking with little water is more yang, and is very strengthening.

Variations: parsnip, onion and cabbage; burdock, swede and cauliflower.

Blanched Salad

1 cup sliced Chinese cabbage
½ cup onion sliced
½ cup carrot thinly sliced
½ cup celery sliced
1 bunch watercress
1-2 pinches sea salt

Put 1-2 inches of water in a saucepan, add salt and bring to the boil. Blanch the vegetables one at a time, starting with the mildest tasting, so that each will keep its distinct flavour. Start by putting the Chinese cabbage in, boil for 1 minute, and remove with a wire mesh scoop or slotted spoon. Next blanch the onion, then the carrot followed by the celery. Last do the watercress for a few seconds only. When each vegetable is removed, spread it out on a dish to cool so that they retain their bright colour.

Mix the vegetables together and add a dressing such as rice vinegar and shoyu or tofu dressing.

Variations: most vegetables can be prepared in this way, for example, green beans, onion and fresh peas, or cauliflower and broccoli.

Pressed Salad

½ lettuce shredded
½ cucumber thinly sliced
½ cup radishes thinly sliced
2 pinches sea salt

Mix the cut vegetables and salt together. They can be pressed in one of three ways, firstly in a commercial salad press, secondly by placing a saucer on the vegetables with a stone or heavy jar on top, and thirdly by repeatedly pressing on them with the palm of your hand. The first two methods take 2-3 hours, the third about five minutes. After pressing, squeeze the excess water from the vegetables, and add rice vinegar or a dressing.

Variations: red radish and cucumber; lettuce, celery and daikon (mouli).

Brine Pickles

½ lb carrots
2 medium onions
1 cup cauliflower
1 cup white cabbage
1 pint water
2 teaspoons sea salt

To make the brine, boil the salt in the water until it dissolves, then allow to cool. Slice the vegetables thinly and pack tightly in a glass or ceramic jar. Add brine to cover the vegetables and put a stone or cup on top to keep them under the surface.

Store in a warm place for 5-10 days, tasting a piece occasionally. When the raw taste is replaced by a sharp, slightly sour taste they are done. Store in a refrigerator or cool place, and enjoy over the next 2 or 3 weeks.

Variations: onion, celery and green beans; pickling onions.

Beans

Aduki Beans

1 cup aduki beans
4 inch piece kombu seaweed
4 cups water
¼-½ teaspoon sea salt or 1-2 teaspoons shoyu

Spread the beans on a flat plate and pick out stones and impurities. Wash in a sieve under a tap. Wipe kombu with a damp cloth and place in the bottom of a saucepan. Add the beans and water and cover, bring to the boil, turn heat to low, and simmer for 1 hour. Add more water if needed to keep the beans covered. Add salt or shoyu and cook 20-30 minutes more. Remove the cover and simmer until all the liquid has gone.

Variations: Just before adding the salt or shoyu, add chunks of carrot and onion, or Hokkaido pumpkin.

Lentils

1 cup green or brown lentils
3 inch piece wakame seaweed
2½-3 cups water
¼ cup chopped parsley or spring onions
¼ teaspoon sea salt or 1-2 teaspoons shoyu

Spread the lentils on a flat plate and pick out stones and impurities, then wash in a sieve under a tap. Wipe the wakame with a damp cloth to remove excess salt, place in a saucepan, add the lentils, then the water. Cover and bring to the boil. Turn heat to low and simmer for 30 minutes. Add salt or shoyu and cook 20-30 minutes more. Remove cover and allow any remaining liquid to cook off. Add parsley or spring onions and serve.

Variations: Diced vegetables can be added just before adding the salt or shoyu, for example carrot and onion or onion and celery.

Chickpeas

1 cup chickpeas
4 inch piece wakame seaweed
3 cups water
¼-½ teaspoon sea salt or 1-2 teaspoons shoyu

Chickpeas are usually pressure cooked to speed up the long cooking time they require. Spread them on a flat plate and pick out the impurities, then wash in a sieve under a tap and soak for 12 hours.

Wipe the wakame with a damp cloth and place in a pressure cooker, followed by the chickpeas and water. Cover, bring to pressure, turn heat to low and cook for 1 ½ hours.

Remove the pressure cooker from the heat and cool by running cold water over it. Remove cover, add salt or shoyu, and simmer 30-40 minutes, by which time all the liquid should have gone.

Variations: Just before adding the salt or shoyu, add diced carrot and onion, or Hokkaido pumpkin. Chopped parsley or spring onions can also be added at the end of cooking.

Chickpea Salad

1 cup chickpeas cooked as above
½ cup celery sliced
½ cup onion sliced
½ cup radishes sliced
1 cup lettuce shredded
2 tablespoons tahini
2 tablespoons rice vinegar
1 teaspoon mustard, freshly ground seeds or powder
2 teaspoons shoyu

Mix the chickpeas and vegetables together. Puree the tahini by slowly adding the vinegar and shoyu, stir in the mustard, and mix into the salad.

Chickpea Pate

1 cup chickpeas cooked as above
1 tablespoon tahini
1 teaspoon mustard, freshly ground seeds or powder
1 tablespoon rice vinegar
1 teaspoon shoyu
¼ cup chopped chives or parsley

Puree all the ingredients together in a suribachi (Japanese mortar) or in a blender. Serve with the chives or parsley as a garnish.

Scrambled Tofu

1 cake of tofu
1 teaspoon sesame oil
¼-½ cup chopped spring onions or parsley
½ teaspoon shoyu

Brush a frying pan with the oil and heat for 1 minute. Add the tofu, breaking it up with a wooded spoon. Cook on a medium heat for 3-4 minutes, turning occasionally. Add shoyu and spring onions and cook 1 minute more, then serve.

Sea Vegetables

Cucumber and Wakame Salad

10 inches wakame
½ cucumber
2 pinches sea salt
2 teaspoons rice vinegar

Wash the cucumber and slice finely. Place in a bowl, add water to just cover and sprinkle on the salt. Leave 30-45 minutes. Quickly wash the wakame to remove excess salt, soak for 10 minutes, then cut into 1 inch pieces. Keep the wakame soaking water for a soup or other dish (as it will contain many minerals). Drain the cucumber and mix with the wakame. Add the rice vinegar and serve.

Variations: Soaked wakame can be included in the ingredients of any pressed or raw salad to add a quite different colour and taste.

Arame

½ cup dried arame
1 medium onion sliced
1 medium carrot sliced or cut in matchsticks
1-2 teaspoons shoyu

Quickly wash the arame in water to remove excess salt. Place in a bowl, cover with water and soak for 10 minutes. Remove the arame and slice into 1-2 inch pieces. Place the onion and carrot in a saucepan, and the arame on top. Add the soaking water and enough additional water to just cover the arame. Cover, bring to the boil, reduce the heat to low and simmer for 30 minutes. Add the shoyu and simmer without a lid until all the water has gone. Mix together only at the end, and serve.

Variations: Burdock or onion and salsify and onion; carrot and roasted sesame seeds or roasted and sliced almonds.

Hiziki

Cook as for arame, but with a longer total cooking time of 50-60 minutes. Hiziki is also excellent when combined with vegetables or roasted seeds or nuts.

Hiziki Salad

½ cup dried hiziki
½ cup onion thinly sliced
½ cup cauliflower thinly sliced
½ cup celery thinly sliced
¼ cup roasted sunflower seeds

Cook the hiziki as above, without any vegetables. Blanch the vegetables as described in the Blanched Salad recipe. Mix the hiziki, vegetables and seeds together and serve. A dressing such as tofu dressing could be added if desired.

Kombu and Carrot Rolls

2 carrots cut into 2 inch pieces
4 inch strip of dried kombu per piece of carrot
6 inch piece of wakame stem or gourd strip per piece of carrot
1-2 teaspoons shoyu

Wipe the kombu with a damp cloth to remove excess salt and soak for 10 minutes or until soft. Roll each piece of carrot in a piece of kombu and tie in the centre with the wakame stem or gourd strip. Arrange all the rolls on the bottom of a saucepan and half cover with water. Cover, bring to the boil, turn heat to medium low and simmer for 20-30 minutes. Add the shoyu and cook 10 minutes more without a lid so that all the water is cooked away.

Variations: You can also try making rolls with parsnips, burdock, salsify or daikon (mouli).

71

Fish

Shallow Boiled Fish

1 plaice fillet
1-2 tablespoons shoyu
1 teaspoon ginger juice squeezed from grated root ginger
1 tablespoon rice vinegar

Wash the fish and marinate in the shoyu, vinegar and ginger juice for 1 hour. Put the fish in a frying pan, add the marinade and enough water to half cover the fish. Simmer on a medium flame for 2-3 minutes, turn over and simmer for another 2-3 minutes or until the fish is cooked all the way through. Serve with a salad or plenty of lightly cooked greens.

If you have less time, instead of marinating the fish you can just add the shoyu, vinegar and ginger juice when it is cooked.

Variations: The same method can be used to cook cod, haddock, flounder, trout and other white fish.

Baked Fish

1 cod fillet
1-2 tablespoons shoyu
¼ teaspoon freshly ground mustard seeds or mustard powder
1 tablespoon rice vinegar

Wash and marinate the fish as above. Place on a baking tray, add the marinade and enough water to half cover the fish. Bake in an oven at 400F (gas mark 6) for 10-20 minutes or until the fish is cooked through.

Instead of marinating the fish you can also bake it straight away, with the shoyu, vinegar and mustard added to it in the baking tray.

Variations: Any white fish can be cooked using this method.

Sauces and Dressings

Kuzu Gravy

2 cups of vegetable cooking water or plain water
¼ cup mushrooms thinly sliced
1 tablespoon kuzu
1-2 tablespoons shoyu

Heat the water in a frying pan, add the mushrooms and shoyu and simmer for 5 minutes. Puree the kuzu in 3 tablespoons of cold water. Remove the pan from the heat and stir in the kuzu. Return the pan to the heat and simmer for 5 minutes, gently stirring to prevent lumps forming. Serve over vegetables, noodles, and other dishes.

Variations: For a different taste add sauteed onions or a little ginger juice squeezed from grated root ginger. (If you cannot find kuzu, use arrowroot instead).

Tofu Dressing

1 cake tofu
¼ onion diced finely
½-1 teaspoon miso
½ teaspoon rice vinegar
¼ cup chopped spring onions, parsley or chives

Puree the miso in 1-2 tablespoons water in a pestle and mortar or suribachi (Japanese mortar). Add the onion and puree it with the miso. Add the tofu and rice vinegar and puree until creamy, adding a little water if necessary. Mix in the spring onions, parsley or chives. Serve on blanched, pressed or raw salads.

Vinegar and Shoyu Dressing

3 teaspoons rice vinegar
1 teaspoon shoyu

Mix the vinegar and shoyu together, and serve over salads or steamed vegetables.

Tahini Dressing

2 tablespoons tahini
1 tablespoon shoyu
¼ onion diced finely

Puree the onion, tahini and shoyu in a pestle and mortar or suribachi. Slowly mix in enough water to make a thin paste. Serve on blanched, pressed or raw salads.

Umeboshi (Pickled Plum) Dressing

2 umeboshi or 2 teaspoons umeboshi paste

Puree the flesh of the plums or the paste with a few teaspoons of water until a thin, smooth paste is obtained. Use on salads and vegetable dishes.

Condiments

Gomasio (Sesame salt)

1 teaspoon fine sea salt
10-20 teaspoons sesame seeds

Roast the salt in a frying pan on a medium heat for 5 minutes, then put into a mortar or suribachi. Roast the sesame seeds in the pan until they become lightly golden and can be easily crushed between two fingers. Stir frequently to get even roasting. If the seeds begin to pop, turn the heat lower. Put the seeds in the mortar or suribachi and grind with the salt until about ⅔ of the seeds have been crushed.

Home made gomasio has a delicious nutty fragrance and taste, and can be sprinkled on grains, breakfast porridge, noodles and vegetable dishes. If it is stored in an airtight jar it will stay fresh for 1-2 weeks. You may well want to make up 2 or 3 times the quantities given above.

Roasted Seeds and Nuts

Seeds such as sesame, sunflower and pumpkin are most easily roasted in a dry frying pan. Nuts like almonds, walnuts, hazelnuts and peanuts may be roasted in a pan, or in an oven which makes even roasting easier.

When roasting in a pan, cook on a medium low heat for 5-10 minutes, stirring frequently to obtain even roasting. When done seeds and nuts are slightly darker in colour, and have a fragrant aroma and taste. A few drops of shoyu can be added a minute before the end of cooking for seasoning.

When roasting in the oven, put the nuts on a baking tray and bake for 5-10 minutes at 400F (gas mark 6), or until they become slightly darker in colour with a fragrant aroma.

Seeds and nuts can be used as snacks, in desserts, or in grain and vegetable dishes.

Desserts

Fruit Jelly (Kanten)

3 sweet apples sliced
2 cups water
3 tablespoons concentrated apple juice
1 pinch sea salt
Agar-agar flakes or powder

Wash and slice the apples, place in a saucepan with the water, juice and salt. Add the amount of agar-agar indicated by directions on the packet (it varies from make to make). Bring to the boil while stirring, reduce heat to low and simmer 5-10 minutes. Rinse a mould with cold water and pour in the fruit. Place in a refrigerator or cool place to harden, then turn out on a flat serving dish.

Variations: Any fresh or dried fruits can be put in this jelly, such as pears, peaches or dried apricots. Dried fruits will need to be cooked 5-10 minutes longer to soften.

75

Baked Apples

Sweet apples
1 tablespoon sultanas per apple
1 teaspoon tahini per apple
1 teaspoon barley malt (malt extract) per apple
1 pinch sea salt

Core the apples from one end only. Mix the sultanas, tahini, malt and salt together in a bowl and fill the apples. Place on a baking tray and bake in the oven at 375F (gas mark 5) for 15 minutes or until soft.

Soya Milk Custard

1½ cups sugar free soya milk
1 tablespoon concentrated apple juice
1 tablespoon kuzu (or arrowroot)
5-6 drops vanilla essence (optional)

Put soya milk, apple juice and vanilla in a saucepan and bring to the boil. Remove from the heat. Puree the kuzu in 2-3 tablespoons cold water and add to the saucepan. Return the pan to a low heat and simmer for 5 minutes, stirring constantly to prevent lumps forming.

More or less kuzu can be added, depending on how thick you like your custard! It is delicious on baked apples, pear and apple crumble, or just on its own.

Rice Pudding

2 cups cooked short or medium grain rice
¼ cup sultanas
3 tablespoons barley malt (malt extract)
1 pinch sea salt
4 cups water

Place all the ingredients in a saucepan and simmer for 30 minutes. Pour into a baking dish and bake at 325F (gas mark 2) for 30-40 minutes. Serve with chopped nuts on top.

Pear and Apple Crumble

2 sweet apples sliced
2 pears sliced
2-3 tablespoons barley malt
1 tablespoon kuzu (or arrowroot)
3 cups rolled oats
1 cup wholemeal flour
3 tablespoons sesame oil
¼ teaspoon sea salt

Put the fruit and ½ cup of water in a saucepan with a pinch of salt and bring to the boil. Remove from the heat. Puree the kuzu in 2-3 tablespoons cold water and add to the saucepan. Replace the pan on a low heat, simmer for 3-4 minutes stirring constantly to prevent lumps forming. Pour into a baking dish.

To prepare the crumble mix the rolled oats, flour and salt, then rub in oil. Warm the malt to make it thinner, and mix with the oats, then spread over the fruit. Bake in an oven at 350F (gas mark 4) for 30-45 minutes.

Variations: Many fruits can be cooked in a crumble, for example apple and blackberries; dried peaches and apricots.

Stewed Fruit

1 lb. fresh sweet apples or ¼ lb. dried apples, pears, apricots or other fruit
1 tablespoon barley malt
1 pinch sea salt
1 tablespoon kuzu (optional)

With fresh apples, remove the cores and slice thinly. Boil in ½ cup water with the salt and malt for 5 minutes. If there is some liquid left, puree the kuzu in 2-3 tablespoons of cold water and add to the apple. Stir constantly until it has thickened, and serve.

With dried fruit soak in a bowl with enough water to cover the fruit for 20-30 minutes, then add fruit, soaking water and salt to a saucepan and simmer until soft. Add the malt 2 minutes before the end of cooking. If there is some liquid left, add the kuzu as described above, and serve.

Oatmeal Raisin Cookies

2 cups rolled oats
½ cup wholemeal flour
2 tablespoons sesame oil
2 tablespoons barley malt
¼ cup raisins
¼ teaspoon sea salt

Simmer the raisins with just enough water to cover them for 5 minutes. Mix rolled oats, flour and salt, then rub in the oil. Add the raisins with cooking liquid and malt, and stir together. Add enough water to make a thick batter. Lightly brush a baking tray with the oil and form cookies ¼-⅓ inch thick on it. Bake at 375F (gas mark 5) for 25 minutes or until golden brown.

Variations: You can use this basic recipe to make many different kinds of cookies, for example walnut and raisin, apple and ginger, or hazelnut and sultana.

Beverages

Three Year Twig Tea (Bancha or Kukicha)

Simmer 1-2 tablespoons of tea with 2 pints of water for 5 minutes. Pour into a cup through a tea strainer. Return the twigs to the pot, add more water and a few more twigs for your next brew. Experiment with the strength that you prefer, some people like this tea weaker and others stronger.

Further Reading

Some books that will give you a greater understanding of yin and yang applied to diet and other aspects of our lives are given below. Those marked with a star are recommended as good introductory books to these subjects.

* **ACID AND ALKALINE.** Herman Aihara. George Ohsawa Macrobiotic Foundation, 1980.

BOOK OF DO-IN. Michio Kushi. Japan Publications, 1979.

* **THE BOOK OF MACROBIOTICS.** Michio Kushi. Japan Publications, 1977.

THE CANCER PREVENTION DIET. Michio Kushi. Thorsons Publishing Group, 1984.

* **FOOD FOR THOUGHT.** Saul Miller. Prentice-Hall Inc., 1985.

HOW TO SEE YOUR HEALTH: BOOK OF ORIENTAL DIAGNOSIS. Michio Kushi. Japan Publications, 1980.

INTRODUCING MACROBIOTIC COOKING. Wendy Esko. Japan Publications, 1978.

* **INTRODUCTION TO MACROBIOTICS.** Oliver Cowmeadow. Cornish Connection, 1987.

MACROBIOTIC CHILD CARE & FAMILY HEALTH. Michio and Aveline Kushi. Japan Publications; 1985.

* **MACROBIOTIC COOKING.** Michele Cowmeadow. Cornish Connection, 1985.

* **MACROBIOTIC DESSERTS.** Michele Cowmeadow. Cornish Connection, 1985.

MACROBIOTICS FOR PREGNANCY & CARE OF THE NEWBORN. Michio and Aveline Kushi. Japan Publications, 1984.

TAO, THE SUBTLE UNIVERSAL LAW AND THE INTEGRAL WAY OF LIFE. Ni, Hua-Ching. Shrine of the Eternal Breath of Tao, 1979.

* **YOUR FACE NEVER LIES.** Michio Kushi. Avery Publishing Group, 1983.

Teachers & Educational Centres

Classes on the theory and practical application of yin and yang, and individual dietary guidance, are given by a number of teachers and centres in Great Britain and Ireland. Please write to the address below for a full list.

The Community Health Foundation
188 Old Street
London ECIV 9BP

Tel: 071-251-4076

If you have any problems with buying any of the foods mentioned in this book, they can be obtained by mail order from the shop below. They also supply foods wholesale, so you may be able to get your local health or wholefood shop to stock them.

Clearspring Natural Grocer
196 Old Street
London. ECIV 9BP

Tel: 071-250-1708

Other Books Published by Cornish Connection

INTRODUCTION TO MACROBIOTICS

Oliver Cowmeadow

A clear and simple introduction to the macrobiotic approach to a natural and healthy way of eating and living. It describes a nutritious and well-balanced diet, with details of which foods to eat and to avoid. It considers the dietary causes of common illnesses, and how a change in diet can be used to prevent sickness. **Paperback, 30 pages, £1.95.**

MACROBIOTIC COOKING

Michele Cowmeadow

This book describes how to prepare delicious, nutritious and well-balanced meals including soups, grains, beans and vegetable dishes, sauces and dressings, pickles, condiments and beverages. There are menu plans for 7 days' meals, and a wealth of information for those preparing wholefood and macrobiotic meals. **Paperback, 64 pages, £3.50.**

MACROBIOTIC DESSERTS

Michele Cowmeadow

Desserts are an essential part of most people's diet. This book contains over 80 tempting and delicious sugar-free recipes, using simple and wholesome ingredients like fruits, nuts, seeds, grains and natural sweeteners. A section on Christmas cooking includes recipes for mince pies, Christmas Cake and Pudding. **Paperback, 58 pages, £2.50.**

FOOD: Nature's Energy Creates You

Peta Jane Gulliver

The theme of this book is the changing of the seasons, and their effect on us and the energies of food. It shows how to choose seasonal foods, including many wild plants, and to celebrate the traditional Celtic festivals eight times a year. Packed with information, 70 delicious recipes, and many attractive drawings. **Paperback, 98 pages, £4.95.**

FOOD CHILDREN ENJOY

Peta Jane Gulliver

This book will give inspiration and support to parents who wish to feed their children on natural wholefoods. It has clear information on how to create a balanced diet for growing children, how to wean babies, and on food based remedies for minor ailments. All this with a wealth of exciting recipes that children really do enjoy! **Paperback, 80 pages, £4.95.**

These books can be ordered from your local bookshop, or obtained directly from the address below. Please add 10% to your order for post and package. Please enquire for details of wholesale terms.

**Cornish Connection, The Coach House, Buckyette Farm,
Littlehempston, Totnes, Devon TQ9 6ND.
Telephone 080426 593.**